KOSHERHEALTH NUTRITION

THE SECRET OF PERFECT HEALTH, UNLIMITED ENERGY AND A MORE MEANINGFUL LIFE

Based upon Rambam, Chassidus, and Traditional Jewish Sources

(Getting Started Series — Part One)

by

RABBI MEILECH LEIB DUBROW

KosherHealth Nutrition
The Secret of Perfect Health, Unlimited Energy and
a More Meaningful Life
(Getting Started Series — Part One)
Rabbi Meilech Leib DuBrow
©July 2018 by Five Gates Society

Published by:
Five Gates Society
Los Angeles, California
Email: rabbidubrow@fivegates.org
Web: www.fivegates.org
ISBN 978-0-9843997-4-1

"I guarantee anyone who conducts himself according to the directions we have laid down that he will not be afflicted with illness all the days of his life until he ages greatly and expires. He will not require a physician, and his body will be complete and remain healthy all his life."
— Rambam

TABLE OF CONTENTS

The Midrash comments: "While Avraham was traveling in Aram Naharayim...he observed the inhabitants eating, drinking and acting frivolously and wantonly. He said: 'I wish to have no part in this land.' When he arrived at the entrance of Tzur, he observed them weeding... cultivating... He said: 'I wish to have my share in this land.' G-d said to him: 'I shall give your children this land.' "

—Breishis Rabbah, 39:8

INTRODUCTION

What the Morning Never Suspected

Imagine waking up every morning, for the rest of your life, knowing that you are sick. Imagine knowing that the good days will become fewer and further between. And the bad days will become more frequent. Imagine the fear, frustration, and hopelessness you would face. Imagine the impact on your family, friendships, your finances, and your future.

That's chronic illness. A world in which we live longer, but poorer lives. It is the world that three out of four of us will inhabit for the last 20 or more years of our lives. Long years spent coping with heart disease, stroke, obesity, diabetes, arthritis, dementia and Alzheimer's, cancer, and depression.

The irony is that it can all be prevented.

An End to Suffering—Guaranteed

Over 850 years ago, Maimonides (Rambam, as he is known in the Jewish world), wrote in his magnum opus of Jewish Law, *Mishneh Torah*, that health is a necessary condition for everyone.

> *"...maintaining a healthy and fit body is an integral part of Divine service"*
> *(Hilchos Deos, 4)*

Yet many people fail attain it. Rambam attributed this failure, and the resulting life spent in chronic pain and suffering, to three bad habits:

- *Satiation*—overeating to the point of weariness and disgust
- *Sedentariness*—lack of physical exercise and laziness
- *Stress*—excessive preoccupation with matters over which we have little or no control

Yet, through ten volumes of medical writings, his monumental *Mishneh Torah* (quoted above), and his foundational work on Jewish philosophy, *Moreh Nevuchim* (*The Guide for the Perplexed*), Rambam set forth the principles—which when diligently applied—could prevent, and even reverse, the pandemic of chronic illness afflicting our world now.

"I guarantee anyone who conducts himself according to the directions we have laid down that he will not be afflicted with illness all the days of his life until he ages greatly and expires. He will not require a physician, and his body will be complete and remain healthy all his life." (Hilchos Deos, 4

The intent of this Getting Started series is to provide you with the knowledge necessary to replace the three "bad" habits with three practices that will help you realize Rambam's guarantee—specifically, in the areas of:

- Nutrition
- Exercise
- Meditation

This small book, *KosherHealth Nutrition*, is the first in the three-part *Getting Started* series.

A Personal Challenge

The *Getting Started* series was motivated, at least in part, by two challenges I received—one from my eldest daughter, Shoshi, and one from my *eishes chayil*, my wife Yehudis.

After one particularly long discussion at our Shabbos table about spiritually-based, health, fitness and healing (more about that later), my daughter declared, "Tatti, this is far too much for anyone to absorb in one meal. Can't you just write down a few basic notes to get someone started."

That challenge alone was sufficient to get me thinking about a "getting started" series. It was my wife's challenge that set me to writing.

When discussing the day's menu with Yehudis, she said with a touch of incredulity, "But I thought that wasn't allowed on our diet." I tried to explain to her the idea of "principle-based experimentation." Dubious might be a benign description of the look I received.

Looks notwithstanding, the two challenges were sufficient to launch the *KosherHealth Getting Started* series.

NOT ANOTHER ONE

You could reasonably ask: why yet another book on Rambam and health?

I would answer first that peoples' intellects and minds differ greatly, each grasping and being affected differently—to the point that many find it difficult to find the benefit of any particular book (see *Likkutei Amarim, Compiler's Forward*, Rabbi Schneur Zalman of Liadi). So its my hope that where previous works on this subject may have failed, this one will succeed.

Second, I would answer that no other book on the subject has been written from perspective of Torahpractic medicine and KosherHealth—a spiritually-infused approach to health, fitness, and healing, based upon the principles set forth by Rambam and other Torah sources, as illuminated by Chabad Chassidus.

KosherHealth's goals are simple—to help you:

- slow aging
- prevent chronic illness
- increase vitality
- reduce stress, and
- reveal your unique life purpose

By the end of this work, you should have a good idea how to:

- Lose significant weight healthfully over a 12 month period, and maintain that weight loss throughout your life;
- Reduce your risk of nutrition-related chronic illnesses like diabetes, heart disease, and cancer, while avoiding malnourishment or eating disorders from overly rapid weight loss fads;
- Make it easy to adjust your diet as needed to increase your vitality

I'm not a big advocate of anecdotal evidence. But "walking the talk" is often offered in place of more formal credentials. Over the past couple years, I've lost and kept off over 40 pounds, almost 20 percent of my initial weight. I find no difficulty cycling 50 or more miles on a Sunday morning, and I recently completed a century (100 mile) bike ride with my daughter, Shoshi. Following Rambam's dietary principles, I eat healthy yet satisfying meals throughout the week. And on Shabbos and Yom Tov, I take pleasure in eating as much challah, red meat, and dessert as I desire.

She opens her mouth with Wisdom, and the teaching of kindness is on her tongue. She anticipates the needs of her household, and the bread of idleness, she does not eat.

Her children rise and celebrate her; and her husband, he praises her: "Many daughters have attained valor, but you have surpassed them all."
—Eishes Chayil, song at the Shabbos Table

AT THE SHABBOS TABLE

House Rules

Our Shabbos table has two rules.

The first rule prohibits discussion about politics, business, movie reviews and competitive sports. We've made exceptions for non-competitive, individual endurance events, especially if they involves cycling (what can I say: I have a personal bias).

The second rule: Come with questions—lots of them. Questions about the week's Torah portion (my grandson's favorite), about Kabbalah, Chassidus, and the halachos of Shabbos, and about health, fitness and healing—are all encouraged.

Among the questions I frequently hear:

Have you heard about the XYZ weight loss diet?

I've tried every diet. I lose a little weight, and then gain it all back. Why?

What about supplements? Do I really need them? They don't have to be kosher, right?

Someone told me that Jews were originally supposed to be vegetarians. Is that true?

Among the answers, you'll inevitably hear one or all of the following mentioned:

- Rambam's teachings on health
- Evidence-based research is slowly catching up to Torah
- Spiritual sources of illness and healing

But before we go there, there's another question: why is diet and nutrition such a big deal?

The Big Deal About Diets

The vast majority (71 percent) of adults in the U.S. are overweight. Nearly 40 percent are clinically obese.

Being overweight or obese has been tied to an increased risk for serious chronic illnesses, including type 2 diabetes, heart disease, respiratory problems, and most major cancers. In fact, obesity is responsible for more preventable deaths in the U.S. than smoking. And the outlook is not good: the Centers for Disease Control (CDC) statistics show that we are getting fatter. Since the weight loss movement kicked off in the early 90s, adult obesity has increased from 15 percent (1990), to 25 percent (2010), to 40 percent (2017).

There are lots of theories about why we are in this sorry state. The most common is that people are overweight because of gluttony (eating too much) and sloth (moving too little). Therefore, what most diets have in common is the belief that if you eat fewer calories, and exercise more, you will lose weight.

The most popular diets add one or more of the following:

- motivating trainers or health coaches
- telegenic doctors
- restrictive meal plans or cardboard-tasting meal replacements
- punishing workouts

Initially, some people do succeed on almost every type of diet: low carb, low fat, low calorie, Paleo, vegan, grapefruit. Research shows that initially the type of diet doesn't make a difference; no matter what the diet, some will lose and some won't.

Unfortunately, most won't keep the weight off. Approximately 80 percent of those who lose weight dieting gain it back, and then some.

Why?

It's not necessarily a lack of willpower. So you can stop blaming yourself.

In truth, its because your own body is sabotaging you. When you lose weight, your *resting metabolism rate* (RMR: how much energy your body uses at rest) slows down. But when you gain weight back, your RMR isn't restored to its previous level at that weight; it stays slow. So most people who lose weight gain it back at a rate of 2 to 4 pounds per year.

That explains, in part, why some people will tout diets long after they've ceased being effective. Their weight gain is slow, and it is easy to deny as temporary.

Natures Have Changed

Every once in a while, one of our more educated guests will point out that if we rely on Torah for nutritional, or other health and fitness advice (as I advocate), we are immediately faced with a dilemma.

In various areas, Halachah (Jewish law) uses the expression "natures have changed." This implies that our physical nature, and therefore the Halachah, has changed somewhat in our day from the way they were in the time of our Sages.

For this reason, Maimonides (*Moreh Nevuchim, 3:14*) and others write that we should not rely on remedies recorded in the Talmud, unless they have been confirmed by medical experts.

Some note that those things that were prohibited in the first place only because of a common danger, such as drinking from water left uncovered overnight because "a snake may have drunk from it and poisoned it," are no longer prohibited because the danger (such as snakes being everywhere) has ceased to be common.

Similarly, any prohibition that the Torah clearly defines in the context of a specific time or place was in the first place not intended to be forbidden permanently.

However, it is a fundamental principle of our faith that "this Torah will never be exchanged," and the eternal applicability of Torah includes the Talmud.

If so, why is medical information dependent upon "time and place" included in the Talmud at all? Why were these remedies written down if they were not intended to remain pertinent throughout the generations?

The answer, and this an essential underpinning of the entire KosherHealth approach, is that the practical side of Torah stems from the spiritual essence of Torah. The spiritual principles, which are the true source of the medical discussions in the Talmud, Rambam, and other Torah sources, are indeed eternal and completely valid in all areas relating to health.

The Torah principles that should guide our dietary choices are the subject of the aptly named *Section 1: Rambam's Principles.*

Take It With a Grain of Salt

But, posits an unsuspecting guest, why not simply rely on science?

Nutrition research often attracts a lot of media attention and catches the public's eye, especially when it claims that such-and-such food or diet prevents (or causes) so-and-so disease.

For example, three decades ago researchers stated that saturated fat causes heart disease. So most people replaced butter in their diets with margarine. Margarine, of course, contains trans fat, which is far more destructive of heart health than butter.

While it is true that nutrition science is making wonderful strides, its conclusions should never be taken for granted and should be treated as tentative at best.

There are at least three reasons for this.

First, modern nutrition science is relatively new—a 20th century creation. The term vitamin wasn't coined until 1912 and the first vitamin, vitamin A, wasn't discovered until a year later. Essential amino acids—the building blocks of proteins, were not identified until the 1930s. The first Recommended Dietary Allowances (RDAs) were established by the National Research Council in 1941. The USDA Food Pyramid wasn't introduced until 1992.

Second, conducting methodologically sound nutrition research is challenging at best. Most such research depends upon study participants recalling and reporting the foods they've eaten in the previous 24 hours. The problem is, most people respond in the way that makes them look as good as possible. They tend to report eating more "good" foods such as meat, fish, vegetables, and fruit, and less "bad" foods such as cakes, cookies, sugar, candies and fats. In one study, participants reported eating less than is necessary to stay alive.

And there are other challenges for nutrition research. When trying to establish a cause and effect relationship between healthy diets and a reduction in disease, many studies simply ignore the fact that people who eat more healthfully also tend to adapt healthier lifestyles, exercise more, have lower body fat, and are less likely to smoke.

The third problem is primarily a result of the first two. There is really no agreement about what makes us fat and how we lose weight.

As I mentioned above, the traditional position regarding what makes us fat is that we are consuming more calories than we are expending.

The problem with this approach is twofold.

First, not all calories are created equal. Some nutrients lead to greater weight gain than others. For example, fat contains nine calories; carbohydrates and protein four calories. This has led to low and reduced fat products and diets which eliminate fats altogether. The problem is, as I will discuss in a later chapter, we need fats.

Second, the same amount of calories can have drastically different impacts on our bodies. Take, for example, carbohydrates. Some carbohydrates are metabolized at higher rates and others more slowly. The higher rates of metabolism provoke a spike in insulin and eventually lead to insulin resistance and chronic illness (think: high fructose corn syrup).

I'll discuss this more in *Section 2: Breaking It Down.*

And then there's the question of how we lose weight.

We are constantly bombarded with news of fad diets, superfoods, fat burners and metabolism igniters. In truth, these are more sales than science. Most fad diets are unfounded, utter nonsense, and even harmful. The authors only cite the research that supports their point of view, even though there is often a vast research literature that refutes it.

I'll talk about this in *Section 3: Putting It Together.*

CAVEAT EMPTOR

The media often declares that a certain food or supplement is great for you, only to refute it a short time afterwards. One day the "experts" say one thing, the next, another. Then other experts will come along with their solution to making it all simpler, purportedly answering the inevitable question: "What the heck should I eat?"

In truth, you should be wary of any headline, or author, that touts a "shocking new answer" to the diet question. It may be a carefully researched study. If so, the researchers themselves will typically conclude with cautions about the limitations of their research. But it may be just another sensational story intended to catch your attention, so that you'll buy another book or supplement, or join the latest rebranded, multilevel marketing meal replacement scheme.

Since this phenomenon is unfortunately so pervasive, it is important to understand the principles of good nutrition, and to take those into consideration when evaluating any new dietary approach or product.

WHAT WE'LL COVER

Which brings us to this first in the KosherHealth—Getting Started series.

In Section 1, we'll explore three simple principles that will help you know:

- How much should you eat?
- Which foods?
- When and how often?
- How to know if you should change your diet?

In Section 2, we apply those Torah principles to specific proteins, carbs, and fats—how much you need of each, which are the best, and worst, and how to tell if you may be deficient. We'll also look at whether or not you should take vitamin and mineral supplements, and how much water you should actually drink (forget the eight 8-ounce glasses a day formula).

In Section 3, we look at the worst ways to lose weight, a simple approach to meal planning, and some guidelines for changing your eating habits.

Finally, in Section 4, I introduce you to "spiritual eating." We'll do a quick review of what it means to "keep kosher." And then we'll look at why.

So, let's get started.

> *"From Moses [of the Torah] to Moses [Rambam] there was none like Moses."*

SECTION 1:
RAMBAM'S PRINCIPLES

RAMBAM AND HIS WRITINGS

KosherHealth is based upon the principles set forth by Rambam over 850 years ago.

Rabbi Moshe ben Maimon, known in the Jewish world by the acronym "Rambam," and to the world at large as "Moses Maimonides," lived in the 12th century and became one of the most prolific and influential Torah scholars of all time. On his gravestone were inscribed the words, "From Moses to Moses, none arose like Moses." Rambam was a Talmudist, Halachist, physician, philosopher and communal leader.

Rambam considered healing a sacred calling. He was concerned with the welfare of all who needed his care, treating Jew and non-Jew, rich and poor, nobleman and peasant alike. He practiced his calling with selfless devotion.

Rambam wrote ten known medical works in Judeo-Arabic, including:

- *The Art of Cure*—extracts and comments on Galen's extensive writings
- *Commentary on the Aphorisms of Hippocrates*—selections from Hippocrates medical writings with Rambam's analysis interspersed
- *Medical Aphorisms of Moses*—over 1500 aphorisms and decried numerous medical conditions
- *Treatise on Hemorrhoids*—which also discusses digestion and food.
- *Treatise on Cohabitation*—recipes for aphrodisiacs and anti-aphrodisiacs.
- *Treatise on Asthma*—general regimens for health, as well as the effect of climate and nutrition on asthma
- *Treatise on Poisons and Their Antidotes*—an early textbook on toxicology
- *Regimen of Health*— a lengthy discourse on healthy living and the mind-body connection.
- *Discourse on the Explanation of Fits*—guidelines for healthy living and the avoidance of overabundance.
- *Glossary of Drug Names*—a materia medica of over 450 drugs in Arabic, Greek, Syrian, Persian, Berber, and Spanish.

Rambam's advice on physical and spiritual health can also be found in his magnum opus of Halachah (Jewish Law), *Mishneh Torah*, and his foundational work on Jewish philosophy, *Moreh Nevuchim—The Guide for the Perplexed.*

In his work of *Medical Aphorisms*, Rambam wrote that health is a necessary condition for everyone. Yet many people are unable to attain it. Rambam attributed this primarily to:

- *Satiation*—overeating and overindulgence
- *Sedentariness*—lack of physical exercise and laziness
- *Stress*—Excessive preoccupation with uncontrollable matters
- *Lack of knowledge*

It is the last of these four—*lack of knowledge*—with which the following sections are concerned, in the hope that it will provide you with the foundation to avoid the first three.

First Principle: Avoid Satiation

Rambam's first principle of nutrition is: *avoid satiation.*

For Rambam, overindulgence in food, or satiation, was one of the three major habits causing illness (the other two being sedentariness and stress).

> *The preservation of health lies in abstaining from satiation... (Regimen of Health, 1)*

It doesn't matter your age or other personal characteristics:

> *The avoidance of overfilling oneself with food is of benefit for all ages and for any body constitution. (Medical Aphorisms of Rambam, Treatise 17)*

And for Rambam, this matter was significant enough to include in the *Mishneh Torah*, his magnum opus of Jewish Law:

> *Overeating is like poison to the body (Mishneh Torah, Hilchos Deos, 4:15)*

Today's Pandemic

Today, it is easy to understand Rambam's concern. Overweight and obesity, the direct result of overeating, are pandemic in the U.S. According to the National Institutes of Health, more than 70 percent of U.S. adults are considered to be overweight or have obesity:

- About 1 in 3 adults are considered to be overweight
- More than 1 in 3 adults are considered to have obesity
- About 1 in 13 adults are considered to have extreme obesity

People who are overweight or have obesity are at increased risk for a host serious chronic illnesses and conditions, including:

- Type 2 diabetes
- Heart disease
- Stroke
- Cancers, including breast, colon, kidney, gallbladder, ovarian, and liver
- Osteoarthritis
- Mental illness such as depression and anxiety

The consequences of overeating, or satiation, are so grave, it led Rambam to write something quite shocking:

All physicians agree that the consumption of a little bad food is less harmful than the consumption of a lot of good and healthy food. (Regimen of Health, 1)

and

Even the best foods, eaten in excess, corrupt one's digestion and this can lead to illness. (Treatise on Asthma, 5:3)

We'll talk about what Rambam means by "bad" food in the next chapter. The point here is simple: don't overeat!

In addition to the increased risk of chronic illness mentioned above, Rambam was concerned about the more immediate problem caused by overeating—poor digestion.

Satiation causes the filling of the stomach and its distention...the stomach cannot digest the food adequately at all, causing weakness, sluggish movement and heaviness from food. (Regimen of Health, 1)

Indigestion might not seem something to be so concerned about, but as Rambam continues:

When the meal is digested poorly in the stomach, inevitably the subsequent stages of digestion are also bad...(Regimen of Health, 1).

That means that in addition to the stomach pain and nausea, you are also likely to experience:

- Gas
- Constipation & diarrhea
- Lethargy

Sound familiar?

Going to Extremes

However, Rambam was also opposed to going to the opposite extreme—that is, following a highly restrictive diet.

> *Any diet which is followed to the extreme, is also difficult to tolerate and detrimental. (Commentary on Hippocrates Aphorisms, 1:4)*

and

> *An excessively restricted diet is even dangerous to healthy individuals. (Commentary on Hippocrates Aphorisms, 1:5)*

As we'll discuss in the chapter, *5 Worst Ways to Lose Weight*, Rambam's concerns about overly restrictive diets are being realized in some of today's most popular diets.

How Much Is Too Much

So it's clear that overeating, and its opposite, is of major concern. But how much is enough?

The classic approaches involve counting calories, controlling portion sizes, or determining the amount of protein, carbohydrates and fat in your meals. The short answer is that all of these approaches are based upon information that has proven to be highly inaccurate.

Rambam's solution? Appetite management.

Basically, you need to stop eating before you reach satiation:

> *It is important to rely on the principle that a person should not satiate his appetite, but should rather stop eating while a little of his appetite remains (Treatise on Hemorrhoids, 1:2)*

Satiation, in the way that Rambam uses it, basically means stuffing yourself. In other words, stop eating before you exclaim, "I cannot eat another bite."

A person should stop eating before food becomes loathsome to him, preferably at a time when most of his lust for food has been satisfied and when only a little desire for food remains. (Treatise on Asthma, 5:2)

It is before that point, the point where you've eaten so much that the food has become detestable, that you should stop.

Physicians have fixed appropriate limits in this matter by saying that a person should stop eating before he detests it, preferably when most of his appetite has been satisfied and only a little appetite remains. (Treatise on Asthma, 5:2)

Interestingly, Rambam suggests a specific means for knowing how much is too much:

Every person should calculate the amount of food that can be easily tolerated and easily digested. This should be done when one is healthy and it should be calculated in the springtime. This amount should be considered one's basic portion. (Treatise on Asthma, 5:1)

Ultimately, Rambam is asking us to distinguish between physical, or "gut," hunger and hedonic, or "head," hunger.

Hunger is normally triggered by declining blood sugar levels, an empty stomach, and even our circadian rhythm. You know that you are physically hungry, gut hungry, when you feel stomach discomfort, have feelings of emptiness, or are experiencing physical or mental weakness.

Head hunger is another matter. Most of us overeat because of a complex of physiological, psychological and cultural issues. Are you bored, experiencing cravings, an emotional need for food, feeling sad and wanting to fill the void, or you need your afternoon pick-me-up of caffeinated soda?

That kind of hunger is driven by habit, culture and even addiction. And that's not the basis for healthy eating.

Interestingly, several studies have indicated that between three and five years of age, we stop eating according to how full we feel. However, as adults, we typically eat until our plates are empty. And those plates have grown larger over the past five decades.

How?

Restaurant serving sizes have grown over the last several decades. This trickled down to serving sizes in our homes, in the size of packaged food portions, and even the size of our plates and bowls.

The end result is that we don't eat because we're hungry. We overeat.

6 Strategies to Avoid Overeating

We'll explore strategies for developing a healthy eating habit in later chapters. For now, here are six quick tips for managing your appetite so that you don't reach satiation.

1. Eat only when you experience one or more of signs of gut hunger: stomach discomfort, feelings of emptiness, or physical or mental weakness.
2. Use smaller dishes: your dinner plate should be the size of a salad plate
3. Spoil your appetite: begin your meal with soup or salad (not water, as we'll discuss in the chapter on hydration)
4. Eat more slowly: it takes 12-20 minutes for a signal of fullness to reach your brain
5. Avoid distracted eating: if you're reading, conversing, or watching TV, you're less likely to notice your stomach signaling that its full
6. Avoid "just this once" or "just one more": set a limit to how much you need to eat or snack, and stick to it

Getting Started Summary

1. Avoid satiation. Stop eating before you become "stuffed."
1. Avoid extremes. Don't eat so little that you are always gut hungry.
1. Eat when you feel physical hunger—stomach discomfort, feelings of emptiness, or physical or mental weakness.

SECOND PRINCIPLE: STRIVE FOR QUALITY

Rambam's second principle of nutrition is: *strive for quality.*

Strive for excellence in the quality of food. (Regimen of Health, I:6)

The obvious question is: what does quality mean? What is good vs bad food?

The answer is, its not simple.

This [knowledge of what makes a food good] is a very beneficial subject and requires knowledge of the nature of all foods of each and every kind. (Regimen of Health, I:6)

Most of us, of course, are neither food scientists nor nutritionists, and we don't possess "knowledge of the nature of all foods."

Rambam's writings are replete with guidelines about specific types of food, such as meat, fish, dairy, bread and vegetables. He also wrote about hundreds of foods for healing. But as we mentioned in our introduction, nature's change, what was "good" in Rambam's time may not be so now.

For example, Rambam did not have to consider chemical fertilizers, genetic modification, or oceanic mercury levels. In addition, foods that were common in Rambam's time may be less available, or not at all, now. We don't even know to which foods certain words refer: Rambam wrote many of his works in Arabic—which were later translated to Hebrew, several European languages, and then English. Much has been lost in translation.

However, as I stated in the introduction, we're looking for Torah principles that are eternal—not specific recipes.

Defining Quality

One thing is pretty clear from Rambam's vast writings: there is currently no single "popular" diet that satisfies all of Rambam's guidelines. Not raw, not vegan, not low protein, carb, or fat, nor even low glycemic, and certainly not gluten-free or Paleo.

There are certain diets that contain components of a "Rambam" diet, such as the *Mediterranean* and *DASH* (heart healthy) diets. But as we'll discuss later, even these two have elements that violate Rambam's three principles.

What we can say definitively is that two keys to Rambam's definition of food quality are nutrient density and digestibility.

Nutrient Density

Nutrient density compares the amount of nutrients—such as vitamins, minerals, and fiber—to the total amount of calories.

Why is an apple "good" and a bag of pretzels "bad?" They both have approximately 100 calories. However, an apple provides fiber, vitamin C and potassium. You get none of those nutrients from pretzels. Or how about watermelon versus a 12-ounce can of soda: both contain approximately 150 calories. Again, watermelon provides fiber and vitamin C. Soda? Its calories are "empty—devoid of nutrients, but full of added sugar.

As a rule, nutrient-dense foods are unrefined or minimally processed, such as:

- Fruits and vegetables that are that are bright or deeply colored
- Whole grains
- Unsalted nuts and seeds
- Fish containing healthy fats and lower levels of mercury
- Lower fat versions of meat, milk, dairy products and eggs

Lower quality foods include:

- Foods that lighter or whiter in color
- Highly processed snack foods
- Refined sugar-sweetened beverages
- Refined (white) grains
- Fried foods
- Foods high in trans fats

Note: don't confuse nutrient-dense with "energy-dense." Often marketed as healthy, energy-dense foods typically contain "empty" calories from refined sugars and unhealthy fats.

While still not common, one food labeling system that rates nutritional quality based upon nutrient-density is Yale University's Overall Nutritional Quality Index (ONQI; sometimes marketed as NuVal).

The ONQI ranking generally requires that a "customary" serving have:

- Total fat <= 13 grams
- Saturated fat <= 4 grams
- Cholesterol <= 60 milligrams
- Sodium <= 480 milligrams

Based upon ONQI, below is a list of 20 of the highest and lowest quality foods (100 being the best possible score):

Highest Quality	Lowest Quality
Broccoli—100	Hamburger (75% lean)—25
Blueberries—100	Coconut—24
Orange—100	Green olives—24
Green Beans—100	Bagel—23
Pineapple—99	Peanut butter—23
Summer squash—98	Sherbet—23
Apple—96	Reduced-fat sour cream—22
Green cabbage—96	Salted, dry-roasted peanuts—21
Tomato—96	Fried egg—18
Mango—93	Diet soda—15
Red onions—93	Pretzel sticks—11
Low-fat milk—91	White bread—9
Fresh figs—91	Salami—7
Grapes—91	Hot dog—5
Banana—91	Cheese puffs—4
Avocado—89	Milk chocolate—3
Atlantic salmon—87	Apple pie—2
Raw almonds and pecans—82	Crackers—2
Unbuttered, unsalted popcorn—69	Soda—1
Canned tuna in oil, drained—67	Popsicle—1

Keep in mind that the ONQI is only one measure of quality, and it is not widely available on food labels. Nonetheless, its criteria and the list above, provide a somewhat consistent means of measuring quality. Certainly better than the more common approach of simply listing calories and % of RDA (the U.S. government's recommended daily allowance).

Digestibility

Nutrient-density is, however, not the only factor that Rambam considered when determining the quality of a food. Also at issue is digestibility.

Digestion—the process of breaking down larger food particles into individual molecules able to squeeze through the wall of your intestines and ultimately into your bloodstream—is a complex process. Your body uses both mechanical and chemical means to digest food. And there is a lot that depends upon you as an individual (more on that later).

The entire process of digestion takes between 24 to 72 hours. Six to eight hours to pass through your stomach and small intestine. Another 24 hours in your large intestine (colon). And then the elimination of undigested food—which usually begins after 24 hours but can take up to several days.

In general, the ease of digestion is based upon the time it takes food to pass from your stomach to small intestine. By food group, the averages are:

- Water and juices: 20-30 minutes
- Fruit, smoothies, soups: 30-45 minutes
- Vegetables: 30-45 minutes
- Beans, grains, starch: 2-3 hours
- Meat, fish, poultry: 3 hours or more

But there is quite a lot of variance within food groups as well, as you can see from the following table:

Foods	Digestion Times
Juices	
Fruit and vegetable juices, vegetable broth	15-20 min.
Blended vegetables and fruit	20-30 min.
Fruits	
Melons	20-30 min.
Citrus fruits and grapes	30 min.
Apples, pears, peaches	40 min.
Vegetables	
Salad: lettuce, tomato, cucumber, bell pepper	30-40 min.
Green leafy: spinach, kale, Swiss chard (cooked or steamed)	40 min.
Broccoli, cauliflower, squash, string bean	45 min.
Root: carrot, beet, parsnip, turnip	50 min.
Starch: potato, sweet potato, yam	60 min.
Grains	
Brown rice, oat, wheat, spelt	1.5 hours
Legumes, Nuts & Seeds	
Lentils, beans, peas, chickpeas	1.5 hours
Soybeans	2 hours
Sunflower, sesame, pumpkin	2 hours
Almonds, cashews, pecans, peanuts, hazelnuts	2.5-3 hours

Dairy	
Skim milk, soft cheeses and cottage cheese	1.5 hours
Whole milk and cottage cheese	2 hours
Hard cheeses	4-5 hours
Fish, Fowl, Meat and Eggs	
Egg yolk	30 min.
Whole egg (with whites)	45 min.
Salmon, trout and other fatty fish	45 - 60 min.
Chicken	1.5 - 2 hours
Turkey	2 - 2.5 hours
Beef, lamb	3 - 4 hours

Rambam never advises eliminating foods that take longer to digest. But he does advise timing your consumption of foods depending on their digestibility. We'll cover that in the next chapter.

Personal Experience, Cultural Custom, and Unmentionables

Looking at nutrient density and digestibility might seem like good ways to judge the quality of a food. But for Rambam, individual differences in constitution, digestion, and age, among other factors, are important as well.

Every person should learn by experience which foods and beverages, and which activities, harm him and from which he should abstain. He should then conduct himself accordingly and choose all that is of benefit to him according to his intellect and refrain from all that which might harm him. He who conducts himself in this manner rarely needs a physician and always remains healthy. (Medical Aphorisms of Rambam, Treatise 17)

One obvious example of learning from experience is to determine which foods cause you discomfort.

It is appropriate to avoid all foods which generate gas… (Treatise on Asthma, 2:2)

and

> *...he should choose food that is good for his nature, that it should not produce gases or thirst but give him pleasure and lightness in that the stools are moderate with a tendency to a little softness—that is good food and he should take it regularly. (Regimen of Health, I:2)*

Rambam also recognized that cultural norms are important.

> *It is not difficult for us (to explain) why many people eat fruits and do not have fever because customs and dispositions have different laws. If for example, a Hindu would eat properly-prepared bread and sheep's meat, he would certainly become ill; and if one of us would constantly eat rice and fish as the Hindus always do, he would certainly become ill. (Regimen of Health, I:13)*

Regarding the quality of food, one of the factors about which Rambam wrote frequently was (I'm sorry; is there a more delicate, but non-technical, way to say this?) pooping .

> *Pay complete attention to the nature of the stool. Do not become constipated; rather lean slightly toward softness. (Medical Aphorisms of Rambam, Treatise 17)*

Personal Taste

Rambam was not unaware of the role personal taste plays in the quality of food. Basing himself, in part, on the following passage in Tanach:

> *"Eat your bread with joy and drink your wine with a merry heart." (Koheles 9:7)*

Rambam wrote:

> *Beverages and foods which are of slightly inferior quality but more palatable are preferable to those which are better quality but are not pleasant tasting... because digestion of pleasant tasting food is better. (Commentary on Hippocrates Aphorisms, 2:38)*

However, as with everything, Rambam advocated moderation:

Don't act like an animal—seeking the most pleasurable in life and nothing else. (Medical Aphorisms of Rambam, Treatise 17)

Picking the Best Foods

As mentioned above, Rambam wrote about hundreds of foods, both for their nutritional and functional (medicinal) quality.

I'll wrap up this chapter with selected quotes from those writings. Keep in mind that when Rambam writes that a food is bad, that doesn't mean that you should eliminate entirely it from your diet. You just need to be aware of its quality and eat appropriately.

[Note: Rambam lived and wrote over 800 years ago. Nutrition science is barely 100 years old. Do you see a pattern here?!]

Where appropriate, I've add some brief comments.

Meat

The best of meats …graze in the meadow. (Regimen of Health, I:7)

Meadow: In this and other writings, Rambam favors meats from free range cattle and fowl over those raised in "mangers" or pens and coops.

The best part …is the front portion and that which is attached to the bone. (Regimen of Health, I:7)

Best parts: These include briskets, chuck, and rib cuts.

Fat is all bad: it satiates but it corrupts digestion, suppresses the appetite… (Regimen of Health, I:7)

Bad fats: Rambam is speaking here about fat from cattle, not fish (see below). There are a few things to notice here: 1) fat is satiating—you get stuffed faster but with fewer nutrients, and 2) fat is bad for digestion—primarily because it is slower and harder to digest. Note that its role as an appetite suppressant is now used in many ketogenic and low carb/high fat diets.

Fish

Fish with small bodies whose flesh is white and firm and has a good taste, and which come from the sea or from flowing rivers...are not bad nourishment, but one should only eat a little thereof. (Regimen of Health, I:9)

Avoid fish with large bodies and salted ones and those which are extracted from bad waters... (Regimen of Health, I:9)

Size: One pundit recently recommended eating only fish that can fit in a frying pan (hopefully, he was not suggesting that only fried fish is healthy). The following list, based upon recent studies of toxicity in fish, including mercury, may be a better guide. Eat these as often as 2 - 3 times per week:

- Salmon
- Trout
- Tuna (light, canned)
- Herring
- Sardines
- Mackerel (canned)
- Tilapia

Fish that you might want to avoid, or eat much less frequently, include albacore, yellowfin and bluefin tuna, and King mackerel.

Bad waters: Around 50% of the fish consumed today, including salmon, are raised in tiny pens containing thousands of fish. Chemicals, like antibiotics and vaccines, disinfectants, and other chemicals used to prevent corrosion of equipment, are common. Equally troubling is the accumulation of fish waste and uneaten food beneath the pens which can degrade the quality of the water.

Dairy

The milk of the cow is also a good nutriment. (Regimen of Health, I:8)

Good and bad milk: In general, Rambam favors consuming cow's milk. However, in several of his writings, he emphasizes that 1) it should be fresh, and 2) it depends upon your reaction to it (see below).

Milk is good for a person in whom it does not sour in his stomach nor become vaporous nor produce swelling. (Regimen of Health, I:8)

Milk products: There were many derivatives of milk about which Rambam wrote, often due to their digestive or functional (medicinal) qualities. Following, I have excerpted two instances where Rambam favored these derivatives.

Cheese which is...white, sweet, and without fat is good. (Regimen of Health, I:8)

All types of butter, fresh or boiled, are not at all bad foods for all people. (Regimen of Health, I:8)

Vegetables

The vegetables which are bad for all people are the following: garlic, onions, cress, radish, cabbage, and eggplant. All of these are bad nutrients for whoever wishes to preserve his health. On the other hand, cucumbers and gourds are less harmful. (Regimen of Health, I:11)

Bad veggies: Rambam seems to source his list of "bad" vegetables here, and in other of his writings, primarily from the Talmud. This is a good example of "nature's have changed." In other words, were Rambam living today, his list of bad vegetables would likely change. As with Rambam's list of fruits (below), I can find no single factor that links these vegetables.

Fruits

In regard to fresh fruits which are the products of trees, there nourishment is generally bad for people, but some are more harmful than others. There are some that are less bad, close to being good, like figs and grapes. (Regimen of Health, I:12)

Tree fruit: I admit to being somewhat surprised by Rambam's opposition to tree fruits. Many are nutrient dense and reasonably easy to digest. Rambam generally favored berries, grapes and figs—even in their dried forms (see below). One could argue that Rambam preferred fruits that had a lower glycemic index (notwithstanding that the actual measurement was not developed until the late 20th century). Berries generally have low glycemic indexes. Figs and grapes have moderate glycemic indexes. However, many tree fruits have lower glycemic indexes. This one remains a mystery to me.

On the other hand, dried fruits such as raisins and dried figs, and nuts such as pistachios and almonds are not bad. (Regimen of Health, I:13)

Nuts: In general, Rambam considered most nuts "good" food. His primary concern was their digestibility, taking up to 3 hours, on average.

Similarly, the consumption of the different types of sweets (fruits) after the meal is very good because it gives the stomach strength to retain the meal and to digest it. (Regimen of Health, I:13)

Timing: We'll discuss food timing and mixing in the next chapter. Even foods that Rambam considered "not bad," he recommended depending upon when— before, during, or after the meal—they were consumed.

Grains

The bread should not be made from refined flour; the flour should be passed through a sieve and its sourness should be perceptible, and one should add a proper amount of salt. But the bread should be made from coarse kernels, unpeeled and unpolished (i.e., whole bran) and its sourness should be noticeable. (Regimen of Health, I:6)

Sourness: Rambam's use of the term "sourness" may be an instance of something "lost in translation." It seems from numerous sources that he is not referring to sour dough, as it is known today. But rather sourness is a mistranslation of the Arabic word for saltiness.

White bread and bread made from refined flour, and pastas, and fried bread..are not good foods (unless they are well digested. (Regimen of Health, I:6)

Everything prepared from wheat flour which was extremely well sifted represents a food which is difficult to digest but very nourishing. (Treatise on Asthma, 3:1)

All sorts of cakes and pastries are bad. All these are extremely difficult to digest and cause constipation. (Treatise on Asthma, 4:8)

Pasta: No surprise here. Don't eat pasta, cakes or pastries—unless you digest them well. And then I would suggest you save them for Shabbos dessert and never eat to satiation (1st Principle).

Special Foods

Wine: Rambam was vehemently opposed to drinking liquids during a meal (as we'll discuss in the next chapter). But as you can see below, he was strongly in favor of drinking wine—even during the meal.

The best of all nutriments or nourishing foods is wine. It is abundantly nourishing, good, thin, and rapidly digested. It assists digestion, and expels superfluities from the pores of the flesh and exerts the urine and the sweat. (Regimen of Health, I:10)

A small amount of wine, such as three or four glasses imbibed at the time the food is being digested and leaving the stomach, is of benefit for the preservation of the health of human beings and an excellent remedy for most illnesses. (Treatise on Asthma, 7:1)

In yet another example of science-catching-up-with-Torah, one recent study of nonagenarians (90 years and older) found that individuals who drank about two glasses of wine a day were 18 percent less likely than non-drinkers to experience a premature death. That's better than exercise, which cut the same risk by only 11 percent (for those who exercised 15 to 45 minutes a day).

Drunkenness: Rambam's only objections to imbibing wine were when it came to drunkenness and youth. Like honey, Rambam opposed wine for children and youth.

The harm done by wine is due to the large quantity imbibed and certainly drunkenness is harmful. (Treatise on Asthma, 7:1)

Honey is good nourishment for the old and bad for the young…(Regimen of Health, I:9)

Honey and wine are bad for children but salutary for the elderly, especially in the rainy season. (Hilchos Deos, 4:12)

Getting Started Summary

1. Strive for excellence in the quality of your food.
2. Quality has nothing to do with the cost of your food.
3. Favor foods that are nutrient dense and easily digestible.
4. Learn from experience: discover what works best for you
5. If you're over 50, drink wine during and/or after your meals.
6. Your food doesn't need to taste bad to be healthy.

Other Resources

As we noted in the beginning of this chapter, determining the quality of food requires a vast amount of knowledge. In order to aid you in the endeavor, we created the **Rambam Diet Checker** (RDC), a free, online app available at kosherhealthfitness.com.

The **RDC** is an easy way to track what and how much you eat of certain foods daily. At the end of day, it provides you with a Total Diet Quality Score. Over time, you can see the direction the quality of your diet is trending, and make adjustments as needed.

THIRD PRINCIPLE: BE CONSISTENT YET FLEXIBLE

After everything you've read so far, you might be ready to make drastic changes in your diet.

Not so fast!

As the Talmud warns:

Changing one's diet results in digestive trouble. (Nedarim 37b)

Rambam states that the Talmud's warning applies whether the change in your diet is either in quantity or quality. In the following passage, he indicates how great the expected "trouble" or illness will be.

If food intake is greatly in excess of the usual, either in quantity or in quality, then it produces a severe illness. You can predict the severity of the illness by the amount of deviation. If the deviation is large, a severe illness is produced; but if the illness-producing deviation is small, the illness will be mild. (Commentary on Hippocrates Aphorisms, 2:17)

To Change or Not to Change?

So does this mean you should never change your eating and drinking habits?

Read the next passage carefully to discover Rambam's response:

A bad but regular eating or drinking habit is farther removed from being dangerous in the pursuit of health than a sudden change from one habit to another, even to a much better one.

Rambam is clear: Changing your eating or drinking habit is not the problem—changing it suddenly is.

In fact, as you'll see in the following passage, you should change your habits from time to time.

In order to maintain one's health in all circumstances, a person should accustom himself to change from habit to habit, but gradually. (Quoting Galen)...It is good for every person to try everything so that when he must do something to which he is not accustomed, it will not seriously harm him.

Therefore a person should not always retain the same habits but should occasionally indulge in their opposites.   (Commentary on Hippocrates Aphorisms, 2:50)

Consistency is important. But so is flexibility.

[Note: One of the best times to vary your diet is on Shabbos and Yom Tov, when we are commanded to derive pleasure from food.]

Eat When Hungry

One the most important areas to which you can apply this "consistent flexibility" is in the timing of your meals—which concerns not only when you eat, but how often, as well as food combining.

Earlier, when discussing Rambam's first principle—avoid satiation—I mentioned that you shouldn't eat until you experience physical hunger.

As it states in Talmud (*Brochos 62b*), "Eat only when you are hungry."

Rambam echoes this in the *Mishneh Torah*:

A person should never eat except when he is hungry nor drink unless he is thirsty. (Hilchos Deos, 4:1)

He repeats this in his *Regimen of Health*, emphasizing that this applies to drinking water as well.

A person should not drink water except after true thirst...(Regimen of Health, 4)

This latter answers one of the most contentious arguments in nutrition: how much and when should drink water—when you are thirsty, or set amounts—e.g., eight 8-ounce glasses a day. We will discuss this further in the next section. However, its clear that Rambam holds the former view.

Interestingly, even though Rambam states clearly and repeatedly that you should eat and drink only when you are hungry and thirsty, respectively, he warns against doing so immediately at the first sign of either:

That is to say, if he is hungry or thirsty he should wait a little because sometimes it may be a false hunger as well as a false thirst…If this subsides, he should not partake of anything. But if the hunger or thirst intensify, he should eat or drink. (Regimen of Health, 4)

And elsewhere:

One should not rely solely on hunger because stomach ailments often have a false sensation of hunger…(Treatise on Asthma, 6:3)

Scheduling Meals

However, Rambam's advice on how often you should eat, or the timing of your meals, might seem to contradict the "eat when you're hungry" advice. In one of his volumes on health, he states:

The most important thing for the conduct of any person (in relation to health) is to prescribe times for nourishment—whether he should eat once, twice, or three time a day. (Medical Aphorisms of Rambam, Treatise 17)

This seems to imply that you should schedule regular times during the day for eating.

In other health writings, Rambam states that you should not have fixed times of the day for eating and returns to his previous position.

One should only eat when the stomach is empty, not like merchants who fix a certain time of day at a certain known hour which never changes as if the meal was an obligatory prayer. (Treatise on Asthma, 6:3)

and

Ingest food only after digestion of the previous meal, or after moderate exercise, or after flatulence from the previous meal has dissipated. (Medical Aphorisms of Rambam, Treatise 17)

So which is it: Do or don't set certain times to eat?

In fact, its relatively simple. Learn from experience.

If you eat when you are physically hungry, over a period of time, you will notice that this occurs with some regularity throughout your day. For example, I don't have a set time for breakfast; but I generally get hungry about 2 to 3 hours after I wake. That's when I eat my breakfast. If I'm doing an early morning bike ride, I may have some carbs before that; but breakfast itself comes later. For me, the same applies to lunch, dinner, and in-between snacks. However, when I'm visiting friends, I accommodate their schedule.

When timing your meals: Be flexible; don't be rigid.

Clearly, the habit Rambam is suggesting contradicts the way most of us conduct ourselves. In many instances, we seem to have little choice. Our lunch times and breaks are set by our employers (or our children's needs)—Rambam's "merchants." But where possible, you should try to eat only when you're physically hungry and only enough to satisfy that hunger, never overeating.

Ultimately, Rambam is saying, it all depends: upon what you eat, the length or brevity of the day, and according to external circumstances.

Frequency of Meals

Rambam wrote not just about when to eat, but how often.

> *Peoples' customs in this regard vary. Most eat in the morning and in the evening but there are others who eat three times a day and a small number who eat only once a day. The general principle to which one should adhere is that healthy, vigorous people can consume all that they need at one time. However, if weak people such as the elderly and those convalescing from illness eat their entire nourishment at one time, they commit a grave offense agains their health. Rather, they should divide their food according to their weakness so as not to decrease their strength. (Treatise on Asthma, 6:1)*

As we noted before, Rambam is advocating that "Every person should learn through experience."

They are very few people today that qualify as "vigorous," able to consume all they need at one meal. Given the prevalence of chronic illness, Rambam would regard most of us as "weak." For us, Rambam advises:

> *Give a weak, elderly person some food three times daily because a weakened body should be nourished in small amounts at frequent intervals. (Medical Aphorisms of Rambam, Treatise 17)*

And elsewhere:

For the elderly, one should feed the body with small amounts at short intervals. (Treatise on Asthma, 6:2)

The key here is to maintain your overall health: not to weaken yourself by eating too frequently or infrequently.

Combining and the Order of Foods

It is not unusual among advocates of certain diets to hear the term "food combining." There are numerous theories about which foods should and should not be eaten together—to say that there is a lack of agreement is an understatement.

Rambam himself wrote on this matter in several of his works:

One should not eat many foods at a single meal...one should eat a single dish per meal, because of the varying digestibility of differing foods. This is also so because then one need not be concerned with the sequence of foods [consumed] because food can impede digestion in many ways. It can impede digestion because of its quality or quantity. (Treatise on Asthma, 5:4)

It is important, however, to understand what Rambam is, and is not, saying here. He is saying that the sequence of foods is important. As we wrote in the previous chapter, various foods have different digestion times. And combining these foods improperly can lead not only to poor digestion, but toxicity.

However, Rambam is not saying that you should eat only one type of food at a meal—meat or vegetables or fruit. Indeed, based upon his writings, KosherHealth advocates including protein, carbohydrates, and healthy fats in every meal.

However, Rambam is advocating minimizing the number of courses you eat at a single meal. And where possible, combining the various foods you are eating at any one meal into a single dish—in order to aid digestion, not to mention prevent overeating.

To guard against satiation, the physicians warned against eating a variety of dishes and suggested that one dish should suffice for each meal so that one should not eat excessively and the appetite subsides before satiation occurs. And he will be spared from the variety of digestions because different foods are digested in different digestions, each food according to its nature. (Regimen of Health, 1)

For example, one of my family's favorite dinners is Lebanese stew: a combination of onion, garlic, olive oil, eggplant, chickpeas, and brown rice. A typical serving—satisfying, but not satiating—contains 10 grams protein, 46 grams carbohydrate, including 9 grams of dietary fiber, and 4 grams of fat. [You'll notice, from the table in the previous chapter, that the major ingredients all have approximately the same digestion time.]

There is one general rule that Rambam provides regarding food combining:

If a person wishes to eat fowl meat and cattle meat together, he should first consume the poultry meat. Likewise, if he desires eggs and poultry meat, he should eat the eggs first. A person should always begin with something light and then proceed to the heavier food. (Hilchos Deos, 4:7)

Rambam also advises:

Consume moist foods in the morning and dry foods in the evening (e.g., bread and meat). Among dry foods are the following three: spices, fruits and vegetables, and meats. (Medical Aphorisms of Rambam, Treatise 17)

One food combination that Rambam seems to advocate against is including fruits with your main meal. Again, in his major Halachic work, *Mishneh Torah*, he writes:

Things which purge the intestines, such grapes, figs, peas, melons, and various types of cucumbers and gourds, should be eaten before the meal. (Kesubos 10b).

Things which bind (constipate) the intestines such as pomegranates, quinces, apples, and small pears, should be consumed immediately after the meal, but one should not eat excessively thereof. (Hilchos Deos, 4:6)

Rambam was also wary of a practice often advocated by so-called weight loss "experts": drinking water just before, during, or even immediately after, your meal.

It is already known to most people that if water is imbibed together with food it counteracts and interposes between the stomach and the food floats and impedes digestion. But if this custom is tolerable to you, drink as little as possible and delay it as much as possible. The best time to drink water is two hours after a meal. (Treatise on Asthma, 7:3)

But in this also Rambam advocates learning from your experience.

The drinking of water after a meal is bad and is harmful to digestion except for one who is accustomed to it. (Regimen of Health, I:4)

Unless you find from experience that drinking a little water with your meal works for you, avoid it.

However, note the words in the first quote, "if this custom is tolerable to you" and in the next, "except for one who is accustomed to it."

If, through experience, you find that drinking a little water immediately after your meal is tolerable or helpful, then go ahead and drink: but "not excessively."

When the food commences to be digested in the intestines, one may drink as much water as one finds necessary. However, even after the food has been digested, he should not imbibe water excessively. (Hilchos Deos, 4:2)

It should also be noted that nowhere in his writings does Rambam advocate filling yourself with water before a meal so that you'll have less room for food. This practice is certainly unnecessary if you follow his first principle: avoid satiation.

Order of Activities

Before leaving the topic of timing your meals, its worth mentioning Rambam's advice regarding eating and exercise.

When a person is hungry, he should not exert himself. (Commentary on Hippocrates Aphorisms, 2:16)

In fact, Rambam generally advocates exercising first and then eating.

If you eat and then exercises, Rambam advises—again as a matter of Halachah that you should minimize movement, even walking excessively, until after the food is fully digested.

When a person eats, he should always be sitting in his place or reclining on the left side. He should not ride or exercise or agitate his body, nor should he promenade, until the food is digested in his intestines. Anyone who promenades immediately after his meal or who fatigues himself brings upon himself serious and grave illnesses. (Hilchos Deos, 4:

Getting Started Summary

1. Eat only when hungry ; drink only when thirsty.
2. Don't be rigid in scheduling when you regularly eat your meals.
3. Eat as frequently as you need to satisfy your hunger and maintain your strength.
4. Minimize the number of courses within a single meal.
5. Combine foods into a single dish.
6. Don't drink water immediately before or after, nor during, your meals Wait until your food is well digested, preferably after two hours.
7. Don't exercise when you're hungry, nor move about excessively immediately after eating.

"*The world can live without wine, but it cannot live without water; the world can live without peppers, but it cannot live without salt.*"
—Jerusalem Talmud, Horeyot 3:5

SECTION 2:

BREAKING IT DOWN

SHOCKING NEWS

Most textbooks on health and nutrition include lengthy sections on macronutrients—protein, carbohydrates, and fats, as well as micronutrients—vitamins and minerals, and hydration.

Popular diets have followed this lead and are often sold as low fat, low carb, or high protein. Even diets that don't mention one of the three macronutrients specifically—such as Paleo, vegetarian, vegan, or gluten free, are often based upon eliminating one or more of these essential foods.

To help you better understand the principles of good nutrition, and to make it easier for you to evaluate any new dietary approach or product—especially those that tout a "shocking new answer" to the diet question—I've put together this next section.

Each chapter of the first three chapters discusses one of the macronutrients. I briefly describe why you need it and then show you how to practically apply Rambam's three principles of quantity, quality, and consistent flexibility. This same approach is then taken in the chapters on vitamins and minerals, and on hydration.

PROTEIN

Don't let anyone tell you otherwise: you need protein in your diet. Lot's of it.

Protein is found in every cell in your body. It is necessary for growth, development, repair, and maintenance of your skin, tissues, organs, muscles, tendons, and bones. Protein is essential to many of your body's processes, such as blood clotting, acid-base fluid balance, immune response, production of hormones and enzymes. Protein foods are also an important source of vitamins and minerals, including vitamins B, D, and E, choline, copper, iron, phosphorus, selenium, and zinc.

Quantity: How much protein do you need?

How much protein you need in your daily diet depends a great deal upon how active you are. While U.S. government guidelines suggest you need only 50 grams of protein a day, a vast amount of research supports much higher amounts—especially if you are physically active—from 1.0 to 2.0 grams per kilogram of body weight per day. The table below gives you some examples of daily protein targets.

Weight (lbs)	Weight (kg)	Daily Protein (g)
125	57	57 - 114
150	68	68 - 136
175	79	79 - 158
200	90	90 - 180
225	102	102 - 204

If you are sedentary, or your regimen consists of less than 30 minutes per day of endurance exercise, you should eat at the low end of this range. If you engage in high intensity intervals or sprints at least once a week, eat in the middle of the range. However, if your regimen includes the full KosherHealth range of RiSE exercises (resistance, intervals, stretching and endurance), consider eating amounts at or near the higher end of the range.

The following table provides protein content for various foods:

Food	Amount	Protein (g)
Meat, Poultry, Eggs		
Chicken, skinless	3 oz	28
Steak	3 oz	26
Turkey, roasted	3 oz	25
Lamb	3 0z	23
Hamburger	3 oz	21
Egg, large	1	6
Fish		
Salmon	3 oz	22
Tuna	3 oz	22
Sardines (canned, in oil)	3 oz	18
Trout	3 oz	17
Tilapia	3 oz	17
Herring	3 oz	15
Dairy		
Greek yogurt	6 oz	18
Cottage cheese (1% fat)	4 oz	14
Regular yogurt (nonfat)	1 cup	11
Milk, skim	1 cup	8
Soy milk	1 cup	8
Mozzarella (part skim)	1 oz	8
String cheese	1 piece	6
Legumes, Grains, Vegetables		
Pinto beans	1/2 cup	11
Lentils	1/2 cup	9
Edamame	1/2 cup	9
Chickpeas	1/2 cup	7
Lima beans	1/2 cup	6

Quinoa	1/2 cup	4
Peas, green	1/2 cup	4
Spinach, cooked	1/2 cup	3
Nuts and Seeds		
Soy nuts	1 oz	12
Peanuts	1 oz	7
Peanut butter	1 tbsp	7
Almonds	1 oz	6
Pistachios	1 oz	6
Walnuts	1 oz	4
Cashews	1 oz	4

Buyer Beware

There are three protein myths that have been promulgated by so-called "experts." Let's get those out of the way now.

Myth 1: Eating a lot of protein leads to chronic kidney disease and increases your risk of osteoporosis.
Fact: There is no significant evidence to support either of these effects if you are otherwise healthy and physically active.

Myth 2: Red meat causes heart disease because of the levels of saturated fat.
Fact: The connection between saturated fat and heart disease has been disproven.

Myth 3: You can get all the protein you need from plants.
Fact: While it is true that a vegetarian diet need not result in a lack of complete amino acids (see below), you'd have to eat a lot of vegetables to get your daily protein requirement, especially if you are physically active. You may have valid personal reasons for not eating meat. However, there is no good Halachic, scientific or health reason to avoid it.

The truth is, increasing the quantity of protein you consume above government recommended levels (i.e., 0.66 grams per kilogram of body weight) has been shown to enhance protein synthesis, postprandial thermogenesis (the rate at which food is broken down and used by your body after a meal), lean body mass, satisfaction, and reduce your cardiometabolic health risk (i.e., your chances of having diabetes, heart disease or stroke).

Quality: What makes a protein good?

As we discussed in the previous section, Rambam defines food quality according to its digestibility and nutritional value.

In order to provide your body with amino acids, protein must be digested—which depends upon its source and the other foods you eat with it. Most animal protein is highly digestible—90 to 99 percent. Plant protein is less digestible—70 to 90 percent; with the exception of soy and legumes, which are over 90 percent digestible.

For proteins, a key factor of their nutritional value is their completeness.

Protein is made up of hundreds or thousands of smaller units, called amino acids, which are linked to one another in long chains. The sequence of amino acids determines each protein's unique structure and its specific function. There are twenty different amino acids that can be combined to make every type of protein in your body. These amino acids fall into three categories:

- *Complete, or balanced, proteins*— are foods which provide adequate amounts of all the essential amino acids. Essential amino acids are required for normal body functioning, but they cannot be made by your body. They must be obtained from food. Of the twenty amino acids, nine are considered "essential." The only source of complete proteins are meat, poultry, fish, eggs and dairy, and soy and quinoa.
- *Incomplete, unbalanced, proteins*—are missing, or do not have enough of, one or more essential amino acids. They do, however, provide nonessential amino acids. Nonessential amino acids can be made by your body from essential amino acids consumed in food or in the normal breakdown of body proteins. Of the twenty amino acids, eleven are considered "nonessential." Plant proteins, such as grains, vegetables, nuts and seeds, and legumes are incomplete proteins.
- *Complementary proteins*—are two or more foods that when eaten in combination form complete proteins. The three most common complementary protein combinations are: grains and legumes; grains and dairy; seeds and legumes

Whether you get your "good" protein from complete or complementary sources, it is important to consume all twenty amino acids daily.

Consistency and Flexibility: How often and when should I eat proteins?

Your experience is an important guide as to what kinds of protein are most agreeable to you.

Recent research, however, suggests that all of your meals and snacks should include protein in some form, especially if you are physically active. Called protein pacing, consuming protein every two hours or so, when combined with a weekly RiSE exercise program, such as KosherHealth, has been shown to improve:

- Physical performance, including upper and lower body strength and endurance, flexibility, and balance
- Body composition, such as weight, waist circumference, body fat percentage, abdominal fat, visceral fat, and lean mass
- Cardiometabolic risk markers, such as systolic blood pressure, blood glucose, LDL, total cholesterol, adiponectin

The research is, of course, not suggesting that you eat steak at every meal. In-between meal snacks, for example, might include high quality energy bars—which typically contain 15 grams of protein from whey or pea isolate. A morning smoothie of Greek yogurt, almond butter, and soy or almond milk (plus the requisite anti-oxidative berries), can also go a long way toward satisfying your daily protein needs.

Remember also to switch things up from time to time. If your in between meal snacks are usually fruit bars, try having cashews and raisins from time to time. For dinner, instead of chicken or fish, try a Lebanese stew or lentil soup.

When Do I Change My Protein Habit?

Protein is everywhere in your body, so there are a wide range of possible symptoms if you're protein deficient. These same signs, unfortunately, can be indicative of other nutritional deficiencies or health problems. Nonetheless, if you experience any of the following, you might check, over a period of 3-4 week days, just how much protein you are getting in your regular diet.

[Note: An easy way to track what you're eating is the **Rambam Diet Quality Scorecard** at kosherhealthfitness.com]

Signs you are getting too little protein may include:

- Low energy levels and fatigue
- Brain fog, poor concentration and trouble learning
- Feeling anxious and moody
- Sleeping poorly
- Muscle, bone and joint pain
- Slow injury recovery, or increased severity of infections and inability to fight infections
- Poor digestion, especially feeling gassy
- Trouble losing weight
- Food cravings, increased appetite
- Irregular menstrual cycle
- Thinning hair, peeling skin, and nail ridges

CARBOHYDRATES

Carbohydrates are your body's main source of fuel or energy. When you eat carbs, you body breaks them down into glucose (blood sugar). Some is used for your immediate energy needs, and the rest is stored in your liver and muscles for later use. All of the cells, tissues, and organs in your body—especially your brain—need glucose. Carbohydrates are important to digestive and heart health, and are also an important source of vitamins and minerals.

Dietary carbohydrates include two types, depending upon their structure:

Simple carbohydrates—or simple sugars, include monosaccharides—glucose, fructose, and galactose; and disaccharides—maltose, sucrose and lactose. Simple sugars are found naturally in fruits, vegetables, and milk. They are also added during food processing.
Complex carbohydrates—or complex sugars, include starches and dietary fiber. There are two types of dietary fiber: soluble and insoluble. Complex carbs are found in whole grain breads and cereals, starchy vegetables and legumes.

Quantity: How much do you need?

How much carbohydrate should be in your diet? That depends upon your:

- Age
- Gender
- Height and weight
- Activity level
- Health and fitness goals

In general, your carbohydrate intake should range anywhere from 40% to 60% of your total caloric intake. That's often hard to calculate, especially on the run. KosherHealth's daily recommendations are :

- Vegetables—4 to 5 servings
- Fruits—3 servings
- Nuts, seeds, and legumes—4 to 5 servings
- Whole grains—2 to 3 servings

Carbs and Exercise

If you are engaging in endurance exercise, such as running or cycling, you need to consume additional carbs during your workout.

In the past, guidelines were usually stated in terms of the amount of carbohydrates you should consume, expressed as grams per hour. For example, the American College of Sport Medicine (ACSM) recommends carbohydrate intake of 30-60 grams per hour. (The guidelines are usually stated in terms of the athlete's body weight, e.g., grams per kilogram of body weight per hour). The problem with this recommendation is that it represents a wide range, and is independent of the type, duration, or intensity of your activity, or training level.

According to more recent studies, it is important to take into account the duration and intensity of your activity, and the source(s) of carbohydrate you consume. Most often, you'll be consuming simple carbs during your workout. You shouldn't be concerned about weight gain, because if you do exercise properly, you're going to burn whatever you consume. But you do need to be concerned about digestion. Your system can only handle so many carbs from a single source before you experience digestive discomfort.

What we now know is summarized in the following table.

Exercise Duration	Amount Needed	Carb Sources
30-75 min.	20g/hour	Single or multiple
1-2 hrs	30g/hour	Single or multiple
2-3 hrs	60g/hour	Single or multiple
3+ hrs	90g/hour	Only multiple

If you're exercising for less than an hour, you don't need much. Even for exercise at a moderate level of intensity, 20 grams of carbohydrate is probably sufficient. That's one Hammer Gel or a packet of Jelly Bellies. However, if you are participating in an endurance event for more than 3 hours, you need multiple types of carbs, such as sucrose and maltodextrin.

Quality: What makes a carbohydrate good?

Not all carbs are created equal.

Good carbohydrates—provide you with a plethora of vitamins, minerals, fiber, and a host of important phytonutrients. The best source of good carbs are unprocessed or minimally processed vegetables, fruits, nuts and seeds, legumes, and whole grains. When choosing foods, prefer those with a higher %DV (percent of daily value) of dietary fiber.

Bad carbohydrates—include refined grains like white bread, pastries, and cookies, candy, and other highly processed or refined foods containing added sugar.

Three important ways to evaluate the "quality" of a carb are:

- Glycemic index or load
- Fiber content
- Nutrient density

I'll discuss each in turn.

Glycemic Index and Load

One way to evaluate the quality of a carbohydrate is by looking at its glycemic index—that's the speed at which it converts to blood sugar. High glycemic index foods rapidly increase your blood sugar and insulin levels, leading to insulin resistance and increasing hunger—which can result in consumption of excess calories and weight gain.

The glycemic index ranges from 0 to 100, with pure glucose having a value of 100. The ranges break down as follows:

0-55 as Low: Carbohydrates that break down slowly during digestion, release blood sugar gradually into the bloodstream, and keep blood sugar levels steady.

56-69 as Medium: Carbohydrates that break down moderately fast during digestion and release blood sugar moderately into the bloodstream.

70-100 as High: Carbohydrates that break down quickly during digestion, release blood sugar rapidly into the bloodstream, causing rapid fluctuations in blood sugar levels.

But you can get a more complete picture of a carbohydrate's effect on your blood sugar when you know not only how fast the food makes glucose enter your bloodstream, but also how much glucose it will actually deliver for a typical serving. That's called a food's *glycemic load*.

For example, watermelon has a relatively high glycemic index of 80. But a typical serving of watermelon has only 6 grams of carbohydrate—so its glycemic load is only 4 (anything below 10 is considered a low glycemic load).

The chart below shows you the glycemic index and load for 50 common foods.

Food	Glycemic index	Serving size (grams)	Glycemic Load
Hummus	6	30	0
Peanuts	13	50	1
Soy beans	15	150	1
Carrots	39	80	2
Chickpeas	10	150	3
Cashews, salted	22	50	3
Grapefruit	25	120	3
Milk, full-fat or skim	31	250 ml	4
Pear, raw	38	120	4
Parsnips	52	80	4
Green peas	54	80	4
Lentils	28	150	5
Apple	36	120	5
Peach	42	120	5
Oranges, raw	45	120	5
Microwave popcorn, plain	65	20	7
Whole wheat bread	69	30	9
Pita bread, white flour	68	30	10

Reduced-fat yogurt with fruit	33	200	11
Corn chips, plain, salted	42	50	11
Banana, raw, average	48	120	11
Grapes, purple	59	120	11
Rye crisps	64	25	11
White wheat flour bread	75	30	11
Apple juice, unsweetened	41	250 ml	12
Orange juice, unsweetened	50	250 ml	12
Potato chips	56	50	12
Honey	61	25	12
Quinoa	53	150	13
Oatmeal	55	250	13
Graham crackers	74	25	13
Gatorade, orange flavor	89	250 ml	13
Brown rice, steamed	50	150	16
Coca Cola® (US formula)	63	250 ml	16
Pretzels, oven-baked	83	30	16
Spaghetti, whole-grain, boiled	42	180	17
Rice cakes	82	25	17
Instant mashed potato	87	150	17
Yam	54	150	20
Instant oatmeal	79	250	21
Spaghetti, white, boiled	46	180	22
Sweet potato	70	150	22
Pizza	80	100	22
Cranberry juice cocktail	68	250 ml	24

Bagel	72	70	25
Spaghetti, white flour	58	180	26
Raisins	64	60	28
White rice, boiled	72	150	29
Baked russet potato	111	150	33

Of course, glycemic index or load is not the entire story. Some foods with high glycemic loads are quite healthy (not pizza, sorry).

Fiber

Important for evaluating the quality of a carbohydrate is its fiber content. There are two types of dietary fiber, and most plant foods contain some of each kind:

- *Soluble fiber* dissolves in water to form a thick gel-like substance in your stomach. It is further broken down by bacteria in your large intestine (colon). Soluble fiber slows digestion and the rate at which carbohydrates and other nutrients are absorbed into your bloodstream. You guessed it—lower glycemic load.
- *Insoluble fiber* does not dissolve in water and passes through your gastrointestinal tract relatively intact and, therefore, is not a source of calories. Insoluble fiber speeds up the movement of food and waste through your digestive system, which helps prevent constipation.

Both soluble and insoluble fiber make you feel full, which can help you eat less and stay satisfied longer. And both types of fiber can be found in a variety of foods, including vegetables, fruits, and nuts and seeds. Soluble fiber is also found in legumes; insoluble fiber in whole grains.

Nutrient Density

We've already discussed nutrient density in the previous section. Let's go a little deeper here.

Plants (think: veggies and fruits) are one of best sources of nutrient dense carbohydrates. More than 25,000 phytonutrients are found in plant-based foods. Phytonutrients, in turn, send information to your genes to control weight, turn metabolism off and on, and prevent every known modern chronic illness.

Here's a list of six types of disease fighting phytonutrients (note the colors):

- *Carotenoids*—act as antioxidants, tackling free radicals that damage tissue, and promoting eye health; (colors) yellow and red—carrots and red pepper—promote eye health; red and pink—tomatoes and pink grapefruit—lower risk of prostrate cancer; green—spinach, kale, swiss chard—protect from cataracts and age-related macular degeneration
- *Ellagic acid*—protects against several types of cancer; found in berries, including strawberries and raspberries, and pomegranates
- *Flavonoids*—including green tea—prevent certain types of cancer; citrus fruits—work as antioxidants reducing inflammation connected with chronic illness; apples, berries, kale, onions—reduce the risk of asthma, heart disease and certain types of cancer
- *Glucosinolates*—contribute to sharp odor and flavor in veggies; may help prevent development and growth of cancer; found in brussel sprouts, cabbage, kale, broccoli

- *Phytoestrogens*—as the name implies, exert estrogen-like effects; soy isoflavones—lower risk of endometrial cancer, lower risk of bone loss in women; lignans with some estrogen-like effects; flaxseed and sesame seeds—may prevent endometrial cancer and osteoporosis.
- *Resveratrol*—acts as an antioxidant and anti-inflammatory, reducing risk of heart disease and certain types of cancer, and extend life; found in grapes, red wine and purple grape juice

Figuring out which foods have the lowest glycemic load, highest fiber, and greatest nutrient density can be a bit daunting (OK, more than a bit). Here are some quick tips:

- Eat the rainbow. In general, the more colors you eat, the more anti-inflammatory, detoxifying, healing compounds you'll get from the phytonutrients your fruits and vegetables provide.
- Keep raw, cut-up vegetables handy for quick snacks— choose colorful dark green, orange, and red vegetables, such as broccoli florets, carrots, and red peppers.
- Add beans (such as garbanzo, kidney, or pinto), lentils, and peas to salads, soups, and side dishes — or serve them as a main dish.

Consistent Flexibility : How often and when should I eat carbohydrates?

Like proteins, the best approach is to have consistent amounts of carbs throughout your day and at every meal and snack. However, two of the most important times to eat carbs are:

1. Morning—Overnight, while you sleep, your body fasts and uses up carbohydrates that it stored away (e.g., glycogen). When you eat carbs first thing in the morning, your body uses those carbs to replenish what you lost overnight.

2. Pre- and post-exercise—Consuming carbs during exercise lasting longer than 90 minutes is needed to prevent hypoglycemia (low blood sugar) and increase endurance capacity (see above).

When Do I Change My Carbohydrate Habit?

Signs that you are consuming too few carbs include:

- Headache
- Weakness
- Fatigue
- Reduced physical performance
- Bad breath
- Muscle cramps
- Heart palpitations
- Constipation or diarrhea

FATS

Fat is essential to your health. Its provides your body with energy, supports cell growth, helps digest, absorb, and transport numerous vitamins, produces important hormones, insulates internal organs against shock, and aids in maintaining your body's temperature. Fat also functions as part of your immune system as a buffer against a host of diseases.

Dietary fat has gotten a bad rap—as evidenced by the plethora of popular low fat diets.

First we need to clarify what we're talking about. There are three major types of dietary fat:

- *Unsaturated fats*—including both mono- and poly-unsaturated fats, which are essential to your health
- *Saturated fats*—found primarily in meat and dairy, and where most of the inaccurate information has been focused
- *Trans fats*—relatively new man-made fats that have no place in your diet

Now let's look at fat through the Rambam's eyes.

Quantity: How much fat do you need?

We've said it before: everyone is different. However, recent research has found that as much as 20 to 35 percent of your calories should come from healthy, or good, fats (see below).

For those of us not big on calorie counting (hand raised), a good rule of thumb is to eat around 0.4 to 0.5 grams of healthy fat per pound of your (target) body weight. For example, if you want to weigh 150 pounds, you could eat as much as 75 grams of healthy fat each day.

Not only do healthy fat-filled meals keep you full, they also burn calories (see below).

Quality: Is there such a thing as good fat?

Like every other type of food, dietary fat contains information and different fats interact with your body in different ways. Whether a fat is good or not depends on the information it communicates. For example, different fats tell your body to either lose weight or gain weight (through a process of binding to special receptors on your cells' nucleus call PPARs).

- Good fats say turn on fat burning genes—improve insulin sensitivity; turn up metabolism.
- Bad fats say turn off fat burning genes—decrease metabolism.

Omega-3 fats, found in kosher fish, are good fats. Monounsaturated fats, found in extra virgin olive oil, nuts and seeds, and avocado, are good fats. Unrefined, polyunsaturated (omega-6) fats are necessary. They are found in natural, expeller or cold-pressed vegetable oils such as grape seed, sunflower, safflower, walnut, and sesame oil.

Here's a list of KosherHealth's most recommended healthy fat sources:

- Fish, such as salmon, trout, tuna, sardines, and canned mackerel
- Eggs
- Olive oil
- Tree nuts, including walnuts, almonds, cashews, pecans and pistachios
- Nut and seed butters
- Avocados
- Edamame
- Dark chocolate (just an ounce)

Most refined polyunsaturated vegetable oils, on the other hand, are bad. They include: refined corn, soy, safflower, and "vegetable" oils.

Trans fats are the worst. They disrupt your metabolism, causing you to gain weight. They are in virtually all processed foods, but sometimes are labeled as hydrogenated or partially hydrogenated oils.

What about saturated fats? Most of the research has focused on saturated dairy fat. And contrary to what we've been told for the past several decades, most recent research indicates that there is no connection between dietary saturated fat and coronary heart disease, stroke, or cardiovascular disease.

Your brain is made up of and needs fat, including a saturated fat called lauric acid (found in mother's milk). Coconuts are a source of saturated fat. Meat and fowl are sources of saturated fat. Eggs, contrary to popular misconception, do not contain a lot of saturated fat. You do not need to avoid saturated fats. Just don't go overboard.

Consistent Flexibility: How often and when should I eat fat?

Good fats can be consumed throughout the day.

The best time to eat meals high in saturated fat is early in the morning; the worst time is late at night. Recent research seems to indicate that saturated fat, especially palmitate (or palmitic acid), affects our cells' circadian rhythm, or internal clock. Palmitate apparently "jet lags" the immune cells that mediate inflammation—causing them to "tell time" inaccurately and increase chronic inflammation. Interestingly, eating good fats—especially omega-3—seems to block this jet lag effect.

When Do I Change My Fat Habit?

Signs that you may have a fatty acid deficiency include:

- Dry, scaly, flaky or lackluster skin
- Dry, lackluster, brittle or unruly hair, and dandruff
- Stiff or painful joints
- Dry eyes, mouth and throat
- Poor wound healing
- Increased susceptibility to infection
- Fatty food craving
- Women only:
    - Inadequate vaginal lubrication
    - Menstrual cramps
    - Premenstrual breast pain/tenderness

VITAMINS & MINERALS

Vitamins and minerals are called *micronutrients* because your body needs relatively small amounts of them. To get adequate amounts, you need food and/or supplements, to prevent deficiencies (see below) and promote optimal health, as well as promote fat loss and muscle gain. Vitamin and mineral deficiencies have repeatedly been shown to be scientifically linked to an increased risk for many dangerous and debilitating health conditions and diseases.

Take Your Vitamins

There are two types of vitamins, water soluble or fat soluble, depending, as their names indicate, whether they dissolve in water or fat.

Water soluble vitamins have many tasks, but one of most important is helping to free the energy in the food you eat. They include:

- B vitamins:
  - Thiamin (B1)
  - Riboflavin (B2)
  - Niacin (B3)
  - Pantothenic acid
  - (B5),
  - B6 (Pyridoxine),
  - Biotin (B7),
  - Folic acid or folate (B9)
  - B12 (Cobalamin)
- Vitamin C (Ascorbic acid)

In general, water soluble vitamins pass from your body (primarily through pish) every few days; so they need to be constantly replenished.

Fat soluble vitamins are essential for maintenance and protection of your body. Fatty tissues and your liver store and release them as needed. They include:

- Vitamin A
- Vitamin D
- Vitamin E
- Vitamin K

Because your body stores fat soluble vitamins, toxic levels can build up—but rarely from food. Toxicity is most likely to happen if you take too much in the form of supplements.

Mineral Water, Anyone?

There are also two types minerals: macro and micro. Your body needs and stores relatively large amounts of macro- (or major) minerals, much smaller amounts of micro- (or trace) minerals. However, both are essential to your health.

Macro-minerals include:

- Calcium
- Chloride
- Magnesium
- Phosphorus
- Potassium
- Sodium
- Sulfur

One of the important tasks of macro-minerals is to maintain the proper balance of water in your body. Other major minerals are responsible for healthy bones. Major minerals are strongly interdependent: having too much of one can cause a deficiency in another. For example: overloading with sodium can cause a loss of calcium; too much phosphorus hampers your ability to absorb magnesium.

All of the micro-minerals normally found in your body could fit into a thimble. Yet they are just as essential as macro-minerals. They include:

- Chromium
- Copper
- Fluoride
- Iodine
- Iron
- Manganese
- Molybdenum
- Selenium
- Zinc

Like macro-minerals, micro-minerals interact with each other, sometimes triggering imbalances. Food is a safe source of micro-minerals; with supplements, you need to be more careful.

Quantity: How much do you need?

The theory is that you can get sufficient quantities of all the vitamins and minerals you need from a healthy diet.

However, the data doesn't bear this out. Take a look at the prevalence of just four common vitamin and mineral deficiencies in U.S. adults:

- Vitamin B6 (80% deficient)—involved in more than 100 enzyme reactions affecting metabolism, brain and nervous system development during pregnancy and infancy, as well as immune function;
- Calcium (68% deficient)—required to maintain strong bones, for muscles to move and for nerves to carry messages between the brain and every part of your body part, and to help release hormones and enzymes that affect almost every function in the human body;
- Magnesium (75% deficient)—essential for many processes in the body, including regulating muscle and nerve function, blood sugar levels, blood pressure, and making protein, bone, and DNA;
- Chromium (90% deficient)—known to enhance the action of insulin, and be directly involved in carbohydrate, fat, and protein metabolism.

These deficiencies are even more common among the elderly, athletes (who have higher vitamin and mineral requirements), and those suffering from malabsorption conditions. A poor diet that relies on junk food, or a diet that lacks adequate fruits and vegetables, can cause serious vitamin and mineral deficiencies.

Difficulty with digestion of food or absorption of nutrients can also result in getting too few of your essential vitamins and minerals. Potential causes of these difficulties include:

- diseases of the liver, gallbladder, intestine, pancreas, or kidney
- surgery of the digestive tract
- chronic alcoholism
- medications such as antacids, antibiotics, laxatives, and diuretics

Vitamin deficiencies can also occur from low or restricted-calorie diets. A recent study analyzing four popular diets found that they were all deficient in vitamins and minerals, ranging from only 22% to 56% deficient. The diets evaluated were Atkins for Life, the South Beach diet, the DASH diet, and the Best Life diet. Analysis showed that each of these four popular diet plans failed to provide even minimum Recommended Dietary Intake (RDI) sufficiency for the 27 micronutrients analyzed. Six micronutrients—vitamin B7, vitamin D, vitamin E, chromium, iodine and molybdenum—were identified as consistently low or nonexistent in all four diet plans. In addition, it was found that in order to meet the minimum RDI requirements, dieters would have to have an average calorie intake of approximately 27,500 calories—more than ten times the daily average for most individuals!

Finally, vitamin and mineral deficiency can also result from an increased need for certain minerals. Women, for instance, may encounter this need during pregnancy, heavy menstruation, and post-menopause.

Quality: Is there such a thing as a bad vitamin or mineral?

The best source of vitamins and minerals is a complete and balanced diet (as recommended in this book), with only a few exceptions. For example, women who dress *tznius* (modestly, according to Halachah, often suffer a vitamin D deficiency. The body makes vitamin D from sunligh)t. If you are covered pretty much head-to-toe, you're not getting much sunlight.

As you'll see from the table below, a varied diet of green leafy vegetables, fish, whole wheat, bananas and berries will provide you with almost everything you need on a daily basis. When the food on your plate falls short and doesn't include essential nutrients like calcium, magnesium, potassium, vitamin D, and vitamins B6 and B12, a supplement can help take up the nutritional slack.

However, dietary supplements are not intended to be a food substitute. They cannot replace all of the nutrients and benefits of whole foods.

Food Sources of 9 Water Soluble Vitamins

Vitamin	Sources
B1—Thiamin	Asparagus, lettuce, spinach, peas, eggplant, soybeans, mushrooms, lentils, black beans, navy beans, pinto beans, sunflower seeds, tuna, whole wheat
B2—Riboflavin	Almonds, spinach, soybeans, mushrooms, eggs, mackerel, whole wheat, yogurt
B3—Niacin	Asparagus, green leafy vegetables, mushrooms, peanuts, corn, sweet potato, carrots, celery, turnips, lentil, barley, brown rice, almonds, peaches, chicken, tuna, salmon,
B5—Pantothenic acid	Avocado, green leafy vegetables, broccoli, split peas, squash, sweet potato, mushrooms, strawberries, sunflower seeds, eggs, whole wheat
B6—Pyridoxine	Avocado, green leafy vegetables, spinach, tomatoes, bell peppers, potato, garbanzo beans, banana, walnuts, peanut butter, sunflower seeds, brown rice, whole wheat, salmon, tuna, trout, chicken
B7	Avocado, green leafy vegetables, carrots, banana, papaya, most nuts, salmon, eggs
B9—Folate (Folic acid)	Avocado, green leafy vegetables, asparagus, broccoli, green peas, black eyed peas, baked beans, lettuce, tomato juice, peanuts, citrus fruits, banana, papaya, whole grains
B12—Cobalamin	Trout, salmon, tuna, eggs
C—Ascorbic acid	Bell pepper, kale, parsley, sweet potato, guava, orange, grapefruit, strawberries, cantaloupe, kiwi, papaya, pineapple, lemon juice

Food Sources of 4 Fat Soluble Vitamins

Vitamin	Sources
A—Retinoids	Green leafy vegetables, carrots, sweet potato, squash, bell pepper, peaches, pumpkin, cantaloupe, beef, eggs
D3—Cholecalciferol	Mushrooms, salmon, mackerel, sardines, tuna, eggs (sunlight)
E—Tocopherol	Green leafy vegetables, tomato, almonds, sunflower seeds, and most other nuts and seeds, blueberries
K	Green leafy vegetables, green beans, green peas, asparagus, broccoli, parsley, carrots, watercress

Food Sources of 5 Macro-minerals

Macro-mineral	Sources
Calcium	Green leafy vegetables, legumes, rhubarb, molasses, sesame seeds, trout, perch, sardines, dairy
Phosphorus	Legumes, nuts and seeds, eggs, fish, whole grains, wild rice
Potassium	Green leafy vegetables, sweet potato, squash, carrots, tomato, banana, peaches, apricots, melon, dates, raisins, prunes, fish
Magnesium	Almonds, bananas, beans, broccoli, brown rice, cashews, egg yolk, fish oil, flaxseed, green vegetables, milk, mushrooms, other nuts, oatmeal, pumpkin seeds, sesame seeds, soybeans, sunflower seeds, sweet corn, tofu, and whole grains
Sodium Chloride (salt)	Legumes, nuts, seeds, whole grains

Food Sources of 9 Micro-minerals

Micro-mineral	Sources
Iron	Green leafy vegetables, broccoli, lima beans, kidney beans, almonds, apricots, raisins, dates, tuna, chicken
Zinc	Green peas, spinach, cashews, sesame seeds, pumpkin seeds, chicken, whole grains
Copper	Green leafy vegetables, navy beens, garbanzo beans, mushrooms, cashews, soybeans, sunflower seeds, molasses, barley
Chromium	Lettuce, onions, tomato, mushrooms, nuts, prunes, brewer's yeast, whole grains
Fluoride	Fish, Water
Iodine	Sea vegetables, green leafy vegetables, asparagus, strawberries, eggs, iodized salt
Selenium	Brazil nuts, walnuts, mushrooms, salmon, whole grains, eggs
Manganese	Green leafy vegetables, berries, pineapple, garbanzo beans, soybeans, spelt, brown rice
Molybdenum	Legumes, whole grains

Consistent Flexibility: How often and when should I eat vitamins and minerals?

If you are eating regular, healthy meals and snacks as recommended throughout this book, then your diet should be sufficient.

The exceptions are the ones mentioned above: the elderly, athletes, vegetarians, and those suffering from malabsorption conditions or on popular diets.

KosherHealth recommends that everyone over 50 years of age take a full spectrum multivitamin (because of their lack of fillers, our favorites are NutraBio Multi-Sport Men's and Women's Formulas—available through Kosher Emporium at the Kosher Health & Fitness website: kosherhealthfitness.com).

If you are taking supplements, see dosage recommendations on the packaging (some supplements need to be taken with meals).

When Do I Change My Habit?

Getting too much of a vitamin or mineral (e.g., toxicity) from your diet is possible, but rare. Toxicity usually occurs with supplement overuse. Following are just a sample of signs that you are overdosing on vitamin supplements.

Signs of Water Soluble Vitamin Toxicity

- Vitamin B3 (Niacin): skin flushing, itching, impaired glucose tolerance and gastrointestinal upset.
- Vitamin B5 (Pantothenic Acid): nausea, heartburn, diarrhea
- Vitamin B6 (Pyridoxine): painful neurological symptoms
- Vitamin C (Ascorbic Acid): kidney stones, excess iron absorption, vitamin B12 deficiency, erosion of dental enamel

Signs of Fat Soluble Vitamin Toxicity

- Vitamin A (Retinoids): nausea, dizziness, fatigue, loss of appetite, dizziness, dry skin
- Vitamin D (Cholecalciferol): elevated blood calcium levels, loss of appetite, nausea, vomiting, excessive thirst and urination, itching, muscle weakness, joint pain, disorientation

Signs of Mineral Deficiency

- Calcium: cramping of the muscles, numbness, tingling in the fingers, fatigue, poor appetite, irregular heart rhythms
- Magnesium: fatigue, muscle weakness or cramping, loss of appetite, numbness, tingling, muscle cramps, abnormal heart rhythms, nausea, vomiting, seizures
- Iron: anemia
- Potassium: muscle weakness or cramping, constipation, bloating, or abdominal pain
- Zinc: loss of appetite, taste or smell

Getting Started QuickTip

Frum Jewish lifestyle encourages modest dress and indoor scholarly activity. As such, it represents a risk factor for vitamin D deficiency, both in men and women. If you are frum, take vitamin D3. Also take magnesium—without magnesium, Vitamin D isn't properly metabolized, making supplementation useless, at best, and unsafe, at worst.

Hydration

There is no question that adequate hydration is essential to your wellbeing. Overall, your body is 70% water, and the water content of your blood, brain, muscles and cells is even higher. On a daily basis, water:

- Regulates body temperature
- Lubricates joints and moistens tissues
- Helps dissolve minerals and nutrients, carrying them to cells
- Protects organs and tissues
- Removes waste and toxins, lessening the burden on kidneys and liver

Quantity: How much water should I drink?

But how much water is enough?

Staying hydrated should be a simple matter. If you're thirsty, drink. As long as you're sedentary, or engaged in light physical activity, that may, in fact, be sufficient.

However, the concept of drinking according to thirst may be too simple to be an accurate if you're more physically active. For years, the message from sports researchers has been that by the time you feel thirsty, you're already dehydrated.

The common wisdom is that most of us don't drink enough water. We are repeatedly told that the average person needs about eight 8 ounce glasses of water per day. But what's average?

Another approach is to consume ounces of water equal to half your weight in pounds. So if you weigh 120 pounds, you should drink 60 ounces of water per day.

But as you might expect, the common wisdom may not be so wise.

According to the drink-when-thirsty advocates, our bodies can handle temporary under-hydration for up to 8 hours. Most endurance runners and cyclists feel thirsty at about two percent dehydration—the point at which performance begins to drop off. Ultra-runners and distance cyclists can maintain performance at three percent dehydration.

Basically, there are three approaches to hydration:

1. Drink enough to satisfy your thirst (KosherHealth recommended).

2. Drink according to a modified formula.

Instead of a generic eight glasses a day, or half your weight, this approach recognizes that you need to modify your hydration according to your activity level and environment. During an activity, you need to consider your sweat rate, the heat and humidity, and how long and hard you are exercising. You also need to consider pre-activity preparation and post-activity recovery.

For example, the American Council on Exercise offers the following guidelines pre-, during, and post- endurance (90+ min) activities:

- 2 - 3 Hours Before: 17 - 20 oz.
- 20 - 30 Minutes Before: 8 oz.
- During: 7-10 oz every 10 - 20 minutes
- After: 8 oz.

3. Drink according to your urine color (I apologize for the yuck factor). You can use the chart on the Kosher Health & Fitness website (kosherhealthfitness. com) to see if you are drinking enough fluids during the day to stay hydrated. But generally, clear or straw colored urine indicates sufficient hydration. By the way, strong smelling urine can also be a sign of dehydration—assuming you haven't eaten asparagus or garlic.

Quality: What's the best way to hydrate?

When it comes to water, you basically have two options: municipal tap water or bottled water. Both are extensively regulated. The health-based standards for both waters are the same for approximately for 80% of the contaminants regulated by each agency.

So what's the difference between the two types of water?

- Regulations: Bottled water is regulated by the Food and Drug Administration (FDA), and tap water by the Environmental Protection Agency (EPA). Some argue that the EPA has tighter restrictions and inspection regimens, while the FDA has a less stringent disclosure of consumer information.

- Environmental Impact: Some research indicates that most purchased plastic bottles are not recycled. Apparently, Americans purchase enough bottled water to circle the globe more than 5 times. Where does it all go?
- Cost: Bottled water is estimated to cost 2,000 times more than tap. Part of this cost is due to the plastic bottle. However, tap water is certainly not free.
- Bottles May Be Harmful: Not all bottles are harmless—some still may contain BPA. And when the bottles are reused, they may release more potentially harmful chemicals and carcinogens. Then again, think about the wonderfully grimy hands that handle your tap water faucets.
- Misinformation: Up to 50% of bottled water comes from the same place as tap water, not from some exotic and pure, picture-perfect mountainous water source. This is easy enough to check.
- Taste: Not to be redundant, but its a matter of taste. Some people are fine with the taste of tap water.
- Pipes: Tap water quality is not just about the municipal water supply. That water also has to travel through your home's plumbing. Lead pipes and plumbing are still relatively common in America, and water testing for the contaminant is notoriously poor. Standard faucet attachments cost about $25 at places like Target or Home Depot, and will remove the vast majority of in-home contaminants. Other filter options include ones that attach to the counter, pipes under the sink, or a water pitcher.

As for other beverages you drink for the purpose of quenching your thirst (as opposed to their nutritional value):

1. Most water substitutes are simply water with something added: herbal tea, sparkling water, spa water.

2. Other beverages that satisfy thirst and supply nutrients include: milk, soy milk, coconut water, kombucha

3. Avoid any beverage which has added sugar or chemicals, including soda and energy drinks

4. Fruit juice is acceptable for both hydration and nutrition once a day.

Its worth mentioning what we discussed in the previous section. Rambam was vehemently opposed to drinking liquids during a meal. However, he was strongly in favor of drinking wine—even during the meal, calling it the "best of all nourishing foods."

And recent research (I love when science-catches-up-with-Torah) that a couple of glasses of wine a day can not only help clear the mind after a busy day, but may actually help clean the mind as well. Recent studies shows that low levels of alcohol consumption tamp down inflammation and help the brain clear away toxins, including those associated with Alzheimer's disease.

Consistent Flexibility: How often should I drink?

Over 200 hundred years ago, the Rebbe Rashab (6th Lubavitcher Rebbe) wrote, "Even mild dehydration reduces blood volume, which reduces blood flow carrying water, oxygen and nutrients to the muscles, organs and glands. Continued loss of water will directly affect the heart and brain, which require large amounts of water and oxygen brought by blood flow."

Other dangers of even mild dehydration include:

- Decreased performance
- Muscle weakness and cramps
- Headache
- Heartburn
- Heart palpitations
- Dizziness
- Overheating
- Irritability

If you find that you are suffering any of the above, especially during moderate to intense physical activity, its time to change your habit.

> *"Changing one's diet results in trouble."*
> —Babylonian Talmud, Nedarim 37b

SECTION 3:

PUTTING IT TOGETHER

Last Week's Cholent

You want to eat healthfully. But you also want to lose weight—as fast as you can.

Well, there are approaches that work, and there are those that should be avoided like last week's cholent.

In this section, we'll look at:

- the five worst ways to lose weight—and we'll name names
- how to put together a simple meal plan based upon Rambam's principles
- a *sage* approach to changing habits

Five Worst Ways To Lose Weight

Despite every thing we've discussed, some of you will be convinced that you need to "go on a diet" in order to lose weight.

OK, I get it.

But if you are going to diet, there are good ways, and some very bad ways.

KosherHealth believes that the best way to lose weight is by following Rambam's three principles:

1.   Quantity: Avoid satiation
2.   Quality: Strive for quality
3.   Habit: Be consistent yet flexible

If your diet follows these three principles, you will:

- Attain a healthy weight over a period of 12 months
- Sustain that weight loss for more than two years
- Find it easy to adjust your diet as needed
- Avoid health risks like malnourishment or overly rapid weight loss
- Reduce your risk of nutrition-related chronic illnesses based like diabetes, heart disease, and certain types of cancer

When combined with the KosherHealth RiSE exercise program, this approach to weight loss works. I personally lost over 40 pounds in less than year and have kept it off for over two years.

That won't stop many from trying a faster approach. People often say to me, "I need a quick start and then I'll eat right."

Most likely, they'll try one of the following types of diets, among which are the five worst ways to lose weight:

1.   Calorie counting
2.   Starvation
3.   Low Fat
4.   Low Carb
5.   YoYo Dieting

Let's discuss each in turn.

Calorie Counting

Calorie counting is the classic approach to weight loss dieting. And as we'll see, its the basis for most other diet practices today, including portion size approaches, point systems, as well as the starvation, low fat and low carb diets discussed below.

Calorie counting is based upon the idea that if you eat fewer calories than you expend, you will lose weight.

In theory, that idea is correct. A pound of body weight is the equivalent of about 3,000 calories. Eat 500 calories a day less than you expend working out or just moving about, and at the end of six days, you should lose one pound of body weight.

In theory. But as a weight loss practice, it is deeply flawed for the following reasons:

1.   It requires time and effort most people are not willing to expend
2.   Label information is not very accurate (5-20%)
3.   All calories are not created equal
4.   The theory is wrong (see *Calorie Counting* below)

<u>Time and Effort</u>

Calorie counting, to work as a weight loss strategy, requires two steps.

First, you have to determine how many calories you actually expend each day, including energy expended for:

- Sleeping
- Personal care (dressing, showering)
- Cooking
- Eating
- Sitting (whether in an office, factory, or your home)
- General household work
- Commuting (by car, bus, cycling)
- Walking at varying paces without carrying anything

- Light leisure activities (chatting, reading a book)
- Working out (aerobic, strength training, stretching)
- Yard work (planting, weeding)
- Housework (sweeping, washing dishes and clothes)
- Childcare

Obviously, the list is as extensive and as varied as your daily activities.

Unfortunately, there is no chart that accurately calculates how many calories you're expending during each activity. Why? Because you also need to take into account your body size and composition, physical activity, as well as your geographic, cultural and economic background.

Think you've got it nailed by using a fitness tracker—such as the Apple Watch or Fitbit Surge?

Think again. A recent study found that even the most accurate tracker was off by an average of 27 percent when it came to measuring energy expenditure. The worst was off by 93 percent!

But let's say you actually come to a reasonable estimate of your daily energy expenditure in calories (be sure to let me know how you did that).

Next, you have to accurately calculate the caloric value of each food you eat. There are, of course, huge government and proprietary databases for doing just that. Unfortunately, none of them seems to agree. For example, we discovered the following disparities while searching three popular food calorie databases:

Item	Lowest (calories)	Highest (calories)
Apple (1 medium)	83	116
Carrot sticks (1 cup)	37	61
Chopped tomato (1 cup)	23	49
Sweet potato (1 large)	231	705
Lean beef (6 oz)	323	506
Bread (1 slice)	51	78

In addition, the caloric value of food is also dependent on the species you eat, how it was cooked, chopped or blended, how much you absorbed, your gut bacteria, and, of course, the accuracy of your portion size estimate.

If this already seems like mission impossible, consider this. How do you accurately estimate the caloric value of multi-item dishes: like a vegetable soup, Lebanese stew, or a fruit, seed, and nut butter smoothie? You can't.

But it gets worse (of course).

Caveat Emptor

The FDA requires companies to display calorie counts on food labels. However, the FDA allows these companies wide latitude regarding the accuracy of those listings—up to 20 percent in either direction. In addition, the FDA doesn't systematically enforce label accuracy, even to that lax degree.

If companies were truly conscientious about food label accuracy, they would have to test the food in a lab, putting a sample of each ingredient in an instrument called a bomb calorimeter. But more often than not, companies simply add up the calories using a standard nutrient database—like the ones discussed above.

However, label inaccuracy is of little consequence, since most of us don't know how many calories we should be consuming in the first place.

A Calorie By Any Other Name

But what if you did know exactly how many calories you are consuming and burning daily?

The counting calories approach still fails.

In the lab, a calorie is the unit of energy required to raise the temperature of one gram of water by one degree Centigrade at sea level. In the lab, all calories burn at the same rate.

But you body is not a lab. In your body, calories are not all the same. Calories from protein, carbs, fat, all send different, complex metabolic signals to your body. Some foods instruct your body to store fat, increase or decrease your appetite, and even speed up or slow down aging.

We've already discussed at length one such instruction: a food's glycemic load. The higher the glycemic load, the faster you absorb a food's sugar, increase blood sugar and insulin levels, and the more that is stored as fat. This in turn leads to insulin resistance, weight gain, increasing cholesterol and triglycerides, fatty liver, and more weight gain.

Think 150 sugar calories from a can of soda versus from homemade vegetable soup.

And how about this for sending mixed signals: There is strong evidence that zero calorie artificial sweeteners can potentially increase your risk for weight gain, metabolic syndrome, type 2 diabetes, and cardiovascular disease. That's because artificial sweeteners can be 1000 times sweeter than sugar. Your body becomes confused and increases insulin production and fat storage. Then your metabolism slows down, you become hungry more quickly, so you eat way more food (especially carbs). Increased belly fat is the inevitable result.

Naming Names

Some of the more popular calorie counting, or low calorie diets include: Medifast/Optavia, NutriSystem, SlimFast, Weight Watchers, Cookie Diet, HMR Program.

Getting Started

The bottom line: calorie counting doesn't work. In fact, a recent study found that people who cut back on added sugar, refined grains and highly processed foods while concentrating on eating plenty of vegetables and whole foods — without worrying about counting calories or limiting portion sizes — lost significant amounts of weight over the course of a year.

1. The kinds of calories you consume has a big impact on how much weight you gain or lose.
2. Whole foods communicate with your body best and most healthfully.
3. If you love sugar, save it for Shabbos and have just a little. Consider it part of "the pleasure of Shabbos."

Starvation Diets

Starvation—restrictive or very low calorie—diets are basically calorie counting taken to the extreme.

They typically consist of meal replacements, such as a liquid shake, a snack bar or a soup, that you consume regularly instead of your regular meal.

If you believe that the reason people are overweight is because of gluttony or sloth, then the obvious way to lose weight is to eat less (exercise optional).

Certainly, Rambam would agree that overeating and being sedentary are two of the three worst habits, contributing to years of illness and suffering. And there are numerous studies that say that we do eat too much and are too sedentary.

So for most people, eating less may in fact be good advice, sort of.

The problem with very low calorie diets is that they are both physically and mentally unhealthy. Not only do they harm your body's metabolism, they can also lead to compulsive and self-destructive eating behaviors.

Most people require 1,800 (women) to 2,100 (men) calories daily to maintain basic health. But most popular starvation diets allow less than 1,500 or even 800 calories. That's less calories than many people expend when they are at rest (e.g., resting metabolic rate, or RMR).

What is your body's reaction to such a low intake of calories?

When your body gets information that it is going through rapid weight changes, and/or not getting all the nutrients it needs, it triggers a genetically coded command to save your life—which is basically, eat more, gain back weight, and store fat in case you find yourself in the same condition in the future.

The short term side-effects of starvation diets include:

- Fatigue
- Digestive issues, including nausea, constipation and/or diarrhea
- Gallstones, often requiring surgical removal of the gall bladder
- Heart problems, including palpitations or arrhythmia
- Loss of lean muscle mass
- Electrolyte imbalances

In addition, numerous studies over the last decade have found very low restrictive diets associated with the onset of eating disorders, including anorexia, bulimia nervosa, and binge eating disorder.

The bottom line: anything taken to the extreme—including restrictive, very low calorie, or starvation—diets not only doesn't work, but is dangerous to your physical and mental health.

Naming Names

Some of the more popular starvation diets include: Medifast/Optavia, SlimFast, 3-Day, Body Reset, Fast Diet, Master Cleanse, Raw Food, Grapefruit Diet, Cabbage Soup Diet, and almost all meal replacement diets.

Getting Started

1.   You need to eat more than your RMR or your body will think that you are starving. In the long run, you will gain back the weight you lost and quite possibly more.
2.   If you want to lose weight quickly, cut out refined and processed foods, eat complete and balanced meals, and engage in moderate-intensity exercise for at least 150 minutes a week (30 minutes per day).

Low Fat Diets

Fat makes you fat. Eat less fat.

So says the U.S. Government (USDA), American Heart Association (AHA), and the American Diabetes Association (ADA), among others. All have recommended low fat diets to prevent and treat obesity, heart disease, and a long list of other chronic illnesses.

It makes sense. And its the very cornerstone of the dietary advice we've been receiving for generations: saturated fats in butter, cheese and red meat cause obesity and clog our arteries.

However, the science doesn't support it.

Americans are in fact eating less fat than they ever have (as a percent of total calories). And yet the rate of obesity is spiraling upward out of control.

We've been taught that eating less fat decreases cholesterol; cholesterol is bad because it causes heart attacks. In fact, high fat diets do not cause heart disease. One famous study showed that people eating a low fat DASH (government recommended heart healthy) diet were dying, while those eating a higher fat Mediterranean diet, including olives, nuts, avocados, and fish, were doing fine.

Some would argue that "nutrition policy has been derailed over the past half-century by a mixture of personal ambition, bad science, politics and bias."

They might argue that pharmaceutical companies want you to believe that "bad" or LDL cholesterol is the single leading factor in the development of heart disease. [In truth, its the ratio of total cholesterol to HDL, "so-called" good cholesterol.] Why? In order to sell more statins—which lower LDL—the biggest selling drugs in history.

Others might say that the food industry makes more money from selling "bad" carbs: fast food, sodas, snacks, and candy bars. And now, more and more of those are kosher—lucky us. In truth, they may simply be following the recommendations of the USDA and the AHA (which, by the way, Procter & Gamble, maker of Crisco oil, helped launch).

Whatever the reason (or conspiracy), the fact is that since the early 70s, we have cut back consumption of saturated fats by approximately 11%, but are now eating a lot more simple carbohydrates—at least 25% more. So instead of eating nutrient rich meat, eggs and cheese, we're eating more pasta, starchy vegetables such as white potatoes, and sugar laden junk food. Indeed, up until 1999, the AHA was still advising Americans to reach for "soft drinks," and in 2001, the group was still recommending snacks of "gum-drops" and "hard candies made primarily with sugar" to avoid fatty foods. After all, soft drinks, fruit juice, muffins, white rice and white bread are technically low in fat.

The bottom line is that we need fat.

Like calories, fats contain information, and different fats interact with your body in different ways. Whether a fat is healthy or not depends on the information it communicates: lose weight or gain weight (through a process of binding to special receptors on your cells' nucleus call PPARs).

- Bad fats say turn off fat burning genes—decrease metabolism.
- Good fats say turn them on—improve insulin sensitivity; turn up metabolism.

Omega 3 fats, as in fish, are good fats. Trans fats are bad. Saturated fats, in moderation, are fine.

Naming Names

Some of the more popular low fat diets include: Ornish, Pritikin, Macrobiotic, TLC.

Getting Started

1.   Eat more omega-3 fats that come from salmon, hearing, sardines, avocado, nuts and seeds
2.   Your brain needs some saturated fat; consider adding lean, red meat to your Shabbos and Yom Tov menu.

Low Carb Diets

You already know the answer to this one: all carbs are not created equal and you need carbs to sustain life.

Low carb diets limit your access to critical phytonutrients found in all plant-based foods, especially fresh, whole and unprocessed foods such as veggies, fruits, nuts, beans, seeds, and whole grains.

As we've already discussed, phytonutrients send information to your genes to: control weight, turn metabolism off and on, and prevent every known modern chronic illness.

In addition, you need fiber (a type of carbohydrate) because it helps you:

- Lose weight
- Lower blood sugar
- Reduce cholesterol

There's not much more I can say about this type of diet that hasn't already been said about calorie counting and low fat diets. They simply don't work in the long run. They're short term weight loss results primarily from calorie restriction.

Enough said.

Naming Names

Some of the more popular low carb diets: Atkins, Dukan, Keto, MIND, Paleo, Ornish, the Zone, South Beach.

Getting Started

1.   Stick to carbs with a low glycemic load: whole, unprocessed fruits and vegetables with lots of fiber.
2.   Eat the rainbow of colors.

YoYo Dieting

It's not a diet per se; its an approach to dieting. It's typically the result of, "I just need a quick start. Then I'll go back to healthy eating."

Repeated dieting leads to weight gain because the brain interprets weight loss diets as short famines and urges you to store more fat for future shortages.

By contrast, the bodies of people who don't diet will learn that food supplies are reliable and they do not need to store so much fat.

People can get into a vicious cycle of weight gain and ever more severe diets—yoyo dieting —which only convinces the brain it must store ever more fat. The research predicts that the urge to eat increases hugely as a diet goes on, and this urge won't diminish as weight is gained back because the brain gets convinced that famines are likely.

Increasingly, evidence suggests that repeatedly losing and gaining weight is linked to cardiovascular disease, stroke, diabetes and altered immune function.

Getting Started

The healthiest way to lose weight is to follow the Rambam's three principles, take it steady and exercise. That is much more likely to help you reach a healthy weight than going on any other kind of diet.

Simple Meal Planning

OK, so now what? How do you turn the last 15,000 words of nutritional wisdom into a simple, daily meal plan?

I personally love bullet lists. If I were making a PowerPoint (or Keynote) presentation, this is what my slides might look like.

Principles

Even if you forget everything else, can't remember all of the lists, tables and tips, remember Rambam's three principles:

- 1st Principle—Avoid satiation
- 2nd Principle—Strive for quality
- 3rd Principle—Be consistent yet flexible

What To Include In Each Meal

Here's KosherHealth's recommendations for what to include in <u>every meal</u>:

- Non-starchy vegetables, especially green leafy and other brightly colored vegetables—as much as you want as long as you don't violate Rambam's 1st Principle
- Nutrient dense, fiber rich, starchy vegetables in moderation (1-2 per day), like sweet potato or squash
- One serving of protein
- If you are eating animal protein: favor eggs, fish, chicken and lean animal meats
- If you prefer a more vegetarian approach, include plant protein such as pea isolate, in your snacks
- One serving of healthy fat in every meal

For your snacks include:

- Low glycemic fruits, especially berries and apples
- Nuts
- Protein bars
- Smoothies

If you're over 50, have one or two cups of red wine in the evening, during or after your meal.

A Daily Plan

Its beyond the scope of this book to provide menus and recipes. The following handful of suggestions are simply to give you some ideas of "getting started" single dish meals (they're ones frequently seen in our household).

Dish	Ingredients
Breakfast	
Protein Smoothie	Greek yogurt, blueberries, strawberries, banana, almond butter, unsweetened almond or soy milk (for desired thickness)
	Supercharge with walnuts, avocado, extra virgin coconut butter, pre-soaked pumpkin, chia, and hemp seeds,
	Taste alternatives: kiwi, ginger, mint leaves, lime

Lunch	Ingredients
Leftover Salad	Leftover protein (e.g., salmon, tuna, chicken, or turkey) from yesterday's dinner, mixed greens, spinach, Romaine, kale, additional veggies (cucumber, tomatoes, carrots, red onion, peas, olives), sliced hard-boiled eggs, dried herbs, raw nuts and/or seeds
	Dressing (select according to taste): extra virgin olive oil, balsamic or wine vinegar, lemon juice, Dijon mustard, salt, freshly ground black pepper, basil, oregano, garlic, turmeric, rosemary
Vegetable Omelet	Eggs, diced tomatoes, green onions, chopped green leafy veggies, kosher salt, fresh ground black pepper, turmeric, olive oil
	Supercharge with low fat or part-skim mozzarella or cheddar cheese
	Taste alternatives: mushrooms, fresh chopped sage, brightly colored bell peppers

Dinner	Ingredients
Lebanese Stew	Pre-cooked chickpeas (garbanzo beans), diced tomatoes, onion, garlic, olive oil, kosher salt, fresh ground black pepper, served over whole grain brown rice
Lentil Soup	Lentils, chopped spinach, onion, garlic, olive oil, basil, oregano, parsley, tomato paste, kosher salt
	Supercharge: whole grain brown rice (instead of noodles)
Squashed Salmon	Salmon fillet, zucchini, yellow and green summer squash, halved cherry or grape tomatoes, kosher salt, fresh ground black pepper
	Side dishes: Swiss chard or kale with onions and garlic, or whole grain brown rice

Some Additional Tips

Also consider the following:

- Reduce your plate size—for your dinner plate use a salad plate
- Avoid processed foods
- Avoid all forms of refined sugars and artificial sweeteners (and all beverages that include them)
- Remove the "avoid" foods from your fridge, home, office, car—anywhere you eat
- If you must indulge in one or two "avoid" foods, do so only on Shabbos and Yom Tov, and only in moderation—don't binge
- If you're over 50, consider taking a high potency multivitamin (we recommend NutraBio)

If you're concerned with food intolerances, such as dairy and gluten, test for them one at at time. When you do, watch for:

- Changes in your digestion (constipation/diarrhea, bloating, gas, reflux)
- Weight gain
- Fluid retention
- Headaches
- Respiratory congestion
- Sleep problems
- Muscle/joints aches and pains
- Changes in your skin (rashes, eczema, acne)

Now, on to the big question: how do you change your eating habit?

CHANGING HABITS

Have you heard any of these?

Did you hear about the seafood diet?
You see food and you eat it.

You're fat and you need to go on a diet.
I'm not going to sugarcoat it because you'll eat that too.

(Paraphrasing Henry Youngman)
My wife/husband is a light eater.
As soon as it's light she/he starts to eat.

How do most people curb their appetite?
At the drive thru window.

This is the one I hear most often

I know what I'm supposed to do, I just can't get myself to do it

The truth? Most of you know how to eat healthfully (hopefully, better after reading this book). And most of you have made one or more of the following resolutions:

- I'm going to eat less
- I'm going to eat healthier
- I'm going on that new [fill in the blank] diet

You told your family and friends about it, posted on Facebook, Twitter and Instagram, shelled out hundreds of dollars for meal replacement bars and shakes that taste more like cardboard than cardboard, and on and on.

The result?

The average person loses 5 to 10 percent of their weight in the first six months, and then regains it back plus more within a couple of years. One study found that after five years, more than 50 percent of dieters regained more than 11 pounds over their starting weight. In fact, several studies indicate that dieting is actually a consistent predictor of future weight gain.

That's no joking matter.

Why do diets so often fail?

Building new habits is hard. We fail because of the following factors:

- *Instant gratification*—most of us want to see significant results now, if not sooner. We get impatient if results don't come quickly. Most people can't sustain a diet for more than 3 months
- *Lack of knowledge*—as much as we know about dieting, few of us know how to build good habits
- *Life is messy*—there are plenty of distractions that can lead us off the "straight and narrow" and right back to our old ways.
- *Bite off more than we can chew*—most of use try to change too many habits at a time. And instead of making small, measurable, changes over time, we make vague, grandiose, and almost impossible to keep resolutions.

The Secret Formula

Around my 20th birthday, I had yechidus (private audience) with the Lubavitcher Rebbe, ob"m. My first of three questions was, "How do I change a bad habit?"

The Rebbe answered with a four-step strategy that has stood by both me and my clients for over 45 years. I call that strategy *The Four Rs: Resolve, Recognize, Remove, and Refocus.*

Resolve: The first step in changing a habit is to know why? Why is this a bad habit for you? What are the consequences of not changing your behavior? You need to know the answer to this question so well that you resolve in your "heart of hearts"—in your innermost being—never to behave that way again.

Lots of people fantasize about building a good habit. But they never clearly answer why they want to change. Excessive fantasizing not only doesn't help your resolve; it can be extremely detrimental. Instead of fantasizing about not eating junk food, visualize eating a handful of almonds and raisins, or a protein energy bar, every day.

Keep in mind: New habits are often very fragile. Your resolve needs to be strong enough to resist the "Forget this, it's not worth the effort!" moments.

Recognize: Next, you need to recognize the situation or circumstances that trigger your bad habit. Common triggers include:

- Time—like a mid-afternoon energy slump
- Location—the kitchen, pantry, office vending machine or lunch room
- Emotional state—feeling bored, sad, or stressed
- Other people—please don't blame it on someone else's lunch
- Preceding events—the long commute to work or home

Remove: Don't rely on willpower. You need to hack your environment—pare down your options so that you don't have a lot of decisions to make about eating healthfully. Making repeated choices depletes your mental and emotional energy, even if those choices are relatively pleasant. Remove junk food from your home, or remove yourself from in front of the vending machine.

Also, its fine to dream big—"I'm going to lose 50 pounds over the next twelve months." It's also important to plan small—"I'm going to lose one pound a week by reducing the size of my dinner plate, or having no cookies, or pastries during the week, but setting aside one treat for Shabbos."

Refocus: Find a substitute for the trigger you recognized above. If certain feelings or times trigger your need to eat, make sure that there are healthy snacks easily available. Make use of your current "bad habit routine" to create a good habit. For example, instead of "I'm going to eat healthier," aim for "When I need a mid-afternoon energy boost, I'm going to eat a high quality energy bar." Or "If its lunch time, I'm going to eat protein and veggies."

Resources for Change

Earlier, I joked about telling your family and friends about your new resolution, or posting it on Facebook, Twitter and Instagram. The truth is, social support is important. Finding a friend or group of friends to build good habits with you is one of the best ways of sticking to it.

On the Kosher Health & Fitness website, we've started Cafe Yadid—a kind of Facebook app, but without the political rants and ruckus cat videos. Its designed specifically for people like you who care that what they put in their body is kosher, and on their body, tznius. People who are passionate about fitness and healthy living—body, mind and soul. People who, whether they're looking for energy bars, supplements, or healthy kosher recipes for a post-workout meal, look not only at the hechsher (kosher certification) but also at the nutrition facts (albeit with a grain of salt).

So if you're looking to share your new habit, or get some help keeping it, check out extrenely undervisited (except by the author) *Cafe Yadid* at kosherhealthfitness.com.

"Within every created thing is an "utterance of G-d's mouth"—the letters of Divine speech that continually brings it into existence—its essence. When your body hungers for a piece of bread, this is a manifestation of your soul's craving for that Divine utterance—the soul of the bread. When you eat the bread and utilize the energy you derive from it to serve G-d, you redeem the Divine within it."
—Rabbi DovBer, Maggid of Mezeritch

SECTION 4:
SPIRITUAL EATING

WHAT IS KOSHER?

[Note: For the vast majority of you reading this book, you not only know what kosher is, you keep kosher. On the other hand, you might be surprised at what you learn.]

What does kosher really mean? What are the health benefits of a kosher diet? Do vitamins and supplements have to be kosher? Does kosher mean the rabbi blessed it?

Most people don't know what kosher means. Those who "keep kosher" for religious reasons typically check for a hechsher (kosher agency certification). Those who aren't frum, think that the definition of kosher is either 1) blessed by a rabbi, or 2) healthier, tastier, or safer (think: allergies or vegan).

None of the above provides a kosher definition nor does it explain why over 90 percent of kosher consumers are not religious Jews.

Kosher Food Trending Hot

Kosher is one of the hottest trends in food. In the U.S. (as of 2015):

- kosher food and beverages account for $17 billion in sales
- over 230,000 products are kosher certified
- 11,000 companies have kosher production facilities
- more than 41% of the country's packaged food and beverage products are labeled kosher

Who is driving this market? Jews make up approximately 2% of the U.S. population, and less than 20 percent of Jews keep kosher. So it's not us.

There are roughly 35 million non-Jewish consumers of kosher food in the U.S. Clearly, the majority of consumers are buying kosher for completely non-religious reasons. Among those reasons (according to a 2014 Mintel survey):

- 55%—health and safety concerns, including avoidance of allergens
- 38%%—vegetarian
- 35%%—taste or flavor
- 16%—rules under which kosher foods are produced, especially purity

Of course, there is nothing particularly healthy about OU-certified candy. And certainly, some kosher-aisle staples have become cross-over hits—like when when Lil' Kim rapped about Moscato wine in 2005, and Bartenura kosher wine became an unexpected favorite for hip hop musicians and their fans.

But is there something deeper here than a food fad based upon misinformation and lyrics of questionable intent?

Defining Kosher

Kosher (or more properly, kashrus) is a system of Jewish religious precepts based upon one verse in Tanach (Bible), extensive discussion in the Talmud, and literally thousands of decisions by Rabbinic authorities over the last 2,000 years and continuing today.

The most literal definition of kosher is fit or appropriate. The term's first and only appearance in the Tanach is in *Megillas Esther (8:4)*, where Esther asks King Achashverosh for permission to rescind Haman's decree, saying, "...if I have found favor in the king's eyes, and the matter is kasher before him [then let Haman's order be rescinded]."

In the Talmud, kosher applies to many different situations besides dietary regulation, including lineage (*Kesubos 13b*), marital status (*Kesubos 23b*), the validity of a sukkah (*Maseches Sukkah*), and an alley's eiruv (*Eiruvin 1:2*).

Kosher Food

However, it is with regard to food that most people are familiar with the term (excluding modern colloquial usage meaning genuine, legitimate, or as slang for cool or chill). In kashrus, there are three key elements:

-
- ingredients—must be inherently kosher or approved as such by a kosher certification agency
- mixtures—may not contain a prohibited combination, such as meat and milk, even if the ingredients are kosher in and of themselves
- equipment—cannot have been compromised by the production of non-kosher foods

Ingredients are also divided into three categories:

- Meat (*fleishig* in Yiddish)
- Dairy (*milchig* in Yiddish)
- Pareve (Yiddish for neutral)

Meat includes all kosher animals and fowl—those that have split hooves and chew their cud—slaughtered in the prescribed manner by a shochet (ritual slaughterer). Examples of kosher animals are bulls, cows, sheep, lambs, and goats. If an animal species fulfills only one of above conditions (e.g., a pig has split hooves but does not chew its cud, or a camel—which chews its cud, but does not have split hooves), then its meat is not kosher. Some fowl may not be eaten, including the eagle, owl, swan, pelican, vulture, and stork. Traditionally kosher birds include goose, duck, chicken, and turkey. Fleishig also includes derivatives from animals and fowl (excluding eggs and milk).

Dairy, to be kosher, must derive from kosher animals. This includes products such as cheese, milk, yogurt, ice cream, etc. Dairy products, of course, also may not contain non-kosher additives, and they may not include meat products or derivatives (for example, many types of cheese are manufactured with animal fats).

All fruits and vegetables, products that grow in the soil or on plants, bushes, or trees, are inherently kosher pareve. However, hybridization of different species—sowing two kinds of seeds in one field or in a vineyard—is not allowed. And fruit from trees planted within the past three years may not be eaten.

Most insects and other invertebrates are forbidden. Consequently, vegetables, fruits and other products infested with such insects must be checked and the insects removed.

Fish and eggs are also pareve. However, only fish with fins and scales may be eaten—tuna, salmon, and herring, for instance. Shellfish such as shrimp, crab, mussel, and lobster are forbidden. Eggs are allowed only if they come from a kosher bird and do not contain blood. Therefore, eggs must be individually examined before use.

Wine and beverages made from grape or grape-based derivatives are kosher only if the grapes come from a kosher winery, under strict rabbinical supervision.

Gelatin, casein, and bull blood (yuck!) are not allowed in the kosher wine-making process. Devices and utensils used for the harvest or the processing of the grapes must be cleansed under rabbinical supervision.

The most well known example of a prohibited mixture is meat and dairy, even when both are initially kosher. The Torah says: "You may not cook a young animal in the milk of its mother" (*Shemos 23:19*). From this, our Sages learned that dairy and meat products may not be mixed together. Not only may they not be cooked together, but they may not be served together on the same table nor eaten at the same time. Even utensils (and equipment) are carefully separated into meat and dairy, and separately labeled. After meat meals, most frum Jews wait six hours before eating dairy. After dairy consumption, many wait one hour.

Kosher law does not distinguish between the status of a finished product and its ingredients. If any part of a product is non-Kosher, the entire product is non-kosher.

Vitamins & Supplements—Kosher?

While this might seem relatively straightforward, the regulations regarding what is and is not kosher can be quite complex (a complete discussion of which is well beyond our scope). Consider, for example, energy bars, a favorite staple of fitness enthusiasts. Most energy bars are a mixture of fruits, nuts and various types of sugar. So basic energy bars pose few kashrus concerns. However, the use of dairy ingredients (such as whey or chocolate chips), or non-kosher marshmallows would compromise the otherwise pareve or kosher status of the bar.

Vitamins and supplements pose additional, yet sometimes subtle, issues. Vitamins are typically divided into two categories, water-soluble—such as vitamins B and C, and fat-soluble vitamins—A, D, E, and K. Each of these pose their own unique kosher issues. But all fat-soluble vitamins share a common problem. In their natural state, fat-soluble vitamins are dissolved in an oil emulsion. Producing a tablet or pill, requires the vitamin be converted into a powdered form. This involves mist spraying the vitamin oil into hot air, and coating them with gelatin to prevent the oil from becoming rancid or oxidizing. Of course, many sources of gelatin are not kosher. (see Rabbi Zushe Yosef Blech, *Kosher Food Production*, "Essays in Kashrus and Food Science: The Story of Vitamins" Wiley-Blackwell, 2nd Edition.)

Additional kosher concerns involve supplements, such as L-Cysteine, an amino acid. L-Cysteine has been used to raise immunity to the flu, and also to treat autoimmune diseases and chronic respiratory problems. L-Cysteine also has the unique ability to maintain healthy lung tissue, support the body's natural defenses and enhance cellular health and longevity. These qualities make L-Cysteine especially beneficial for fitness enthusiasts, the elderly, and those exposed to polluted environments.

However, L-Cysteine has historically been extracted from feathers, pig bristles, and human hair. It is the kosher status of these raw materials that can be problematic. For example, human hair is inherently kosher. But when L-Cysteine first came to market, it was harvested from cadavers—a decidedly non-kosher source. Feathers and pig bristles would initially seem to be cause for concern, but their processing often negates these concerns. (see Blech, op. cit. "The Story of L-Cysteine")

Kosher Symbols

Given the complexity of kosher laws, in concept and practice, most people rely upon kosher certifying agencies—of which there are more than 300 in the U.S. (and over 1,300 worldwide). The largest kosher certification agencies in the United States, known as the "Big Five," certify more than 80 percent of the kosher food sold in the US. They include the OU, OK, KOF-K, Star-K, and CRC.

Kosher certification may be granted by any Rabbinic authority—which has led some to believe that kosher certification is simply a matter of a "rabbi giving his blessing." But as Rabbi Blech points out (op. cit.), "the complexities of modern food production demand specialized expertise in both Halachic (Jewish law) and technical arenas."

Because the business of kosher certification is a huge industry (billing hundreds of millions of dollars annually), it has attracted a large number of individuals and organizations. Knowing what standards are employed by these agencies, and to what level of reliability, poses the kosher consumer with another level of complexity. Therefore, the ultimate advice when in doubt is to "consult your local Rabbinic authority."

1.   When in doubt, check the hechsher (certification). Other than fresh produce, never rely "What could be non-kosher about…" For example, many products—both kosher and non-kosher—contain magnesium stearate, a saturated fatty acid found in many foods and oils. Magnesium stearate, sounds like a chemical, but is often derived from animal sources.

2.   Do not rely on the ingredients list on food labels. What may seem insignificant, can be quite significant for kashrus. For example, carmine, an insect-derived red food coloring that comes from ground up cochineal bugs is often listed as Natural Red 4 or simply "added color." In addition, the FDA allows ingredients that are present only in small quantities to be listed simply as "artificial flavor," "natural flavor," or "spices." But these may be derived from non-kosher sources.

3.   Know your certification agency. Does your level of kashrut observance match up with the koshering agency? Agencies can differ in terms of:

- the kashering process between non-kosher and kosher products run on the same line.
- The ingredients used (e.g. gelatin)
- the frequency of mashgiach (inspector) visits
- Transparency, i.e., how easy is it to find out what leniencies the kosher certification agency follows.

The Kabbalah of Kosher

The previous chapter answered the question, "What is kosher?"

But you might still have the question, "Why keep kosher?"

Most observant Jews keep kosher because G-d said so—its a *mitzvah* (commandment). For others, who grew up in a Jewishly observant (but not necessarily Orthodox) home, it's what feels normal. And then there are those who keep kosher as a way to preserve tradition or their personal identity. "Jewish" food is a part of their family traditions, holiday celebrations, and day-to-day life.

In fact, the mitzvah to keep kosher is a *chok*—a supra-rational commandment, beyond logic. However, essentially all mitzvos are supra-rational. They are the will and wisdom of G-d, and as such transcend human comprehension. The sole purpose of any mitzvah is the fulfillment of a Divine desire.

Nonetheless, as Rambam writes:

> *Although all the chukkim of the Torah are supra-rational decrees... it is fitting to contemplate them, and whatever can be explained, should be explained.*

So how should we contemplate kosher? What of it can and should be explained?

For the answer to that, it helps to know a little Kabbalah.

Hidden Energy

It is written: "Man does not live on bread alone, but by the utterance of G-d's mouth does man live" (*Devarim 8:3*).

Rabbi DovBer, the Maggid of Mezritch, explained the deeper meaning of this verse as follows.

> *Within every created thing is an "utterance of G-d's mouth"—the letters of Divine speech that continually brings it into existence—its essence. When your body hungers for a piece of bread, this is a manifestation of your soul's craving for that Divine utterance—the soul of the bread. When you eat the bread and utilize the energy you derive from it to serve G-d, you redeem the Divine within it.*

This, explains the Maggid, is also the deeper meaning of the verse (Tehillim 107:5), "The hungry and thirsty, in them does their soul envelop itself." When you desire food, you may only sense your body's hunger. However, in truth, "enveloped within" your physical hunger is your soul's hunger for the "soul" of the food— the "sparks of holiness" within it.

The Maggid echoes the Arizal, who taught that when you utilize something for a G-dly purpose you reveal its spark, manifesting and realizing the purpose for which it was created.

No existence is devoid of a Divine spark—nothing can exist without the pinpoint of Divine utterance that imbues it with being and purpose. Every object, force and phenomenon in existence has a Divine spark. This spark embodies its function within G-d's overall purpose for creation.

But all physical substances have a kelipah (shell) that encases and conceals the Divine spark at its core. When you use something to serve G-d, you penetrate its kelipah, revealing and realizing its Divine essence.

Each of us has sparks scattered about in the world for which we are responsible. As you move through life, from place to place, you connect with the sparks waiting for you to release and reveal them.

Eating the Divine

However, not every Divine spark can be released from its kelipah. Certain sparks are inaccessible to us. The fact that something is forbidden by the Torah means that its kelipah cannot be penetrated, so that its spark remains concealed within it and cannot be connected with its Divine source.

For example, when you eat a kosher piece of meat or an energy bar, and use its energy to perform a mitzvah, you reveal the Divine spark within it, connecting it with its Divine source. That allows you to tap into and use unlimited Divine energy.

However, if you do the same thing with meat or energy bars that are not kosher, no such connection occurs. No matter how hard you try, or how you think or feel about it, consuming something non-kosher is an express violation of the Divine Will. You cannot connect with the Divine when you are willfully acting against It.

This is what the Torah means when it uses the terms *assur* and *mutar*—as, for example, when they are applied to kosher and non-kosher food, respectively. Assur is commonly translated as forbidden—but it literally means bound—implying that the Divine sparks within it are are bound within their kelipah and inaccessible to you. Mutar, usually translated permitted, actually means unbound and accessible. From something mutar, you can extricate the Divine sparks, connect them with their Source, and derive unlimited Divine energy from them.

So in the food you eat, there is both materiality and spirituality.

Food's materiality provides life for your body—the substances it needs to produce blood and grow. The food's spirituality—its Divine spark—provides life for your soul.

The way you eat determines whether the food will nourish only your body, or your soul as well.

Eating is pleasurable. And often we eat to satisfy our hunger. But if you only eat for physical survival and pleasure, your existence is limited to the natural and temporary. This kind of eating does not connect to the spiritual dimensions of the food. It is basically "animal" eating—even if you are vegan.

One of the simplest ways to access food's spirituality, and to release the Divine sparks within, is by reciting a blessing and keeping in mind that you are eating "for the sake of Heaven"—to have strength to serve G-d through Torah and mitzvos. When you make a blessing on food, you acknowledge G-d as the source of both the food's physicality and spirituality. You infuse a potentially animal act with awareness of G-d.

The Baal Shem Tov teaches that when you recite G-d's name in the blessings over food, you awaken the Divine Name invested in the food. By eating kosher food, you come in contact with, and release, the Divine sparks meant specifically for your soul.

Only when you are aware of and look beyond food's materiality can you release the Divine sparks imbedded within it. This impacts not only the quality of the food you eat, but the quantity as well.

These acts of G-dfulness (not mindfulness) transform the act of eating into a way to increase the world's consciousness of G-d, bringing about its ultimate redemption.

"Man does not live by bread alone, but by the utterance of G-d does man live."
—Devarim 8:3

BACK AT THE SHABBOS TABLE

DESSERT

By the time dessert is being served at our table, the conversation has ranged far and wide, with a fair amount of Jewish geography, stories, and Torah insights.

Most questions have been answered, although there is always a lot more to discuss than can be covered in a single meal.

The same is true of any book on nutrition. This one in particular only scratches the surface, and is intended, as its title implies, for getting started.

So while you dig into your cherry chunk soy ice cream and homemade brownies, let's do a quick review.

Our physical natures, environments, and even foods to which we have access may have changed over the last 2,000 years. Yet the health and nutrition principles set forth in the Torah are eternal and remain the best guide for making your dietary choices.

While nutritional science can provide some insights into your understanding of how to apply those Torah principles today, you should be wary of any headline, or author, or doctor, that touts a "shocking new answer" to the diet question.

Rambam's three principles provide the answers to our most important dietary questions:

Q: How much should you eat?
A: Avoid satiation. Don't stuff yourself—stop eating while you still have room for more. But don't go to extremes, eating so little that you are always gut hungry.

Q: Which foods should you eat?
A: Strive for quality. Build your diet around nutrient dense and easily digestible foods. Learn from experience which foods and beverages work best for your constitution, digestion, age, culture and circumstances.

Q: When and how often should you eat?
A: Eat when you feel physical or "gut" hunger—stomach discomfort, feelings of emptiness, or physical or mental weakness.

Q: How do you know if you should change your diet?
A: Be consistent yet flexible. Change your diet only gradually. Vary the particular foods you eat to overcome nutritional deficiencies and acclimatize yourself to possible changes in your dietary circumstances.

Everybody and every body needs proteins, carbohydrates, and fats, as well as vitamins, minerals, and water, to function. Let your experience be your guide as to what kinds of each are most agreeable to you. As a general rule, the less processed and more varied your food is, the better.

The worst diets are usually the ones that severely reduce or eliminate an entire food group or restrict your consumption. Avoid "quick start" weight loss diets—if it isn't sustainable in the long run, you shouldn't be doing it in the short run. The healthiest way to lose weight is to follow the Rambam's three principles, take it steady, and exercise. That is much more likely to help you reach a healthy weight than going on any other kind of diet.

Always remember: In the food you eat, there is both materiality and spirituality. Food's materiality provides your body with the substances it needs to live and grow. It's spirituality—its Divine spark—provides life for your soul.

By eating kosher food "for the sake of Heaven," you are performing acts of G-dfulness that increase the world's consciousness of G-d, bringing about the world's ultimate redemption.

Bless and be blessed.

ABOUT THE AUTHOR

Rabbi Meilech Leib DuBrow is the founder of the Five Gates Society and Kosher Health & Fitness. He is the foremose expert on traditional Jewish medicine, from which he compiled Torahpractic healing. Rabbi DuBrow is a nationally recognized educator and public speaker on Jewish health and fitness, as well as Jewish meditative practices, Chassidus and Kabbalah. He is the author of *Jewish Healing for Body & Soul*, *Jewish Healing Practices: The List*, and *350 Healing Light Meditations: Daily Wisdom From Kabbalah*. He runs an active health and fitness coaching practice online and in Los Angeles, California.

Rabbi DuBrow's speaking career spans almost fifty years, and includes a diversity of topics and audiences. He has briefed U.S. generals on the acquisition of parts for fighter jets, the invasion of small Caribbean islands and military arms for Israel. He has advised Congressmen on the pitfalls of export subsidies, Presidents on the futility of sanctions, and local governments on the virtues of the Internet. Rabbi DuBrow has persuaded farmers to sell "cookies not corn," venture capitalists to invest in high tech startups, and sedentary seniors to exercise. He is a frequent speaker on the Kabbalah of healing, the spirituality of fitness, and the secret to building a lasting relationship. As an author, educator, and speaker, Rabbi DuBrow is nationally recognized for making the complex simple, the boring exciting, and the impossible practical.

Rabbi DuBrow not only "talks the talk" but "walks the talk." He is an avid cyclist—regularly cycling over 100 miles per week (and sometimes in a day). His favorite and most common cycling companion is his daughter, Shoshi, and his 11-year old grandson, Mooki (who can out-climb both of them on any ride).

If you want to arrange for Rabbi DuBrow to speak at your event, please contact him directly at rabbidubrow@fivegates.org.

ABOUT TORAHPRACTIC HEALING

Our tradition, and especially Chabad Chassidus, teaches us that together with the healing of physical ailments, a Jewish healer must also help his or her client discover the spiritual source of the ailment. For both client and healer, the goal is "a healthy soul in a healthy body."

Until recently, finding a Jewish healer knowledgeable in both the physical and spiritual functioning of the human body was difficult at best. However, for the past 40 years, Rabbi Meilech Leib DuBrow—who trained as both a rabbi and a holistic health practitioner and master herbalist—has been compiling just such knowledge from classical Torah sources such as Talmud, Kabbalah, Chassidus and Halachah.

The result of that effort has been the development of the Five Gates system of Torahpractic™ healing. Rabbi DuBrow describes Torahpractic healing "as the systematic application of Torah principles to the promotion of health and wellbeing", and says that it specifically "focuses on the spiritual and behavioral corollaries of physical ailments."

Citing the ancient yet highly relevant wisdom of Kabbalah, Rabbi DuBrow explains that the source of health is our connection with the Divine. Healing is about restoring that Divine connection.

To learn more about Torahpractic healing
visit us at:
kosherhealthfitness.com

www.ingramcontent.com/pod-product-compliance
Lightning Source LLC
Chambersburg PA
CBHW060505280326
41933CB00014B/2869